Contemporary Issues in Psychological Assessment

Series Editor
Randy W. Kamphaus
Georgia State University College of Education
Atlanta, Georgia
USA

More information about this series at http://www.springer.com/series/7353

Meghan C. Stiffler • Bridget V. Dever

Mental Health Screening at School

Instrumentation, Implementation, and Critical Issues

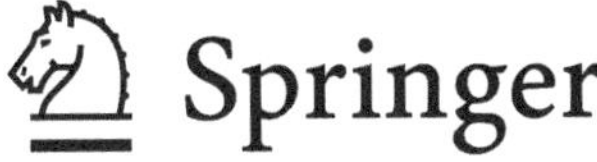

Meghan C. Stiffler
6019 Majestic Pines Drive
Kingwood, TX 77345
USA

Bridget V. Dever
Lehigh University
111 Research Drive
Bethlehem, PA 18015
USA

Contemporary Issues in Psychological Assessment
ISBN 978-3-319-19170-6 ISBN 978-3-319-19171-3 (eBook)
DOI 10.1007/978-3-319-19171-3

Library of Congress Control Number: 2015942137

Springer Cham Heidelberg New York Dordrecht London

Printed on acid-free paper

Springer International Publishing AG Switzerland is part of Springer Science+Business Media (www.springer.com)

To JJ, Patrick, and Baby Girl—You inspire me each and every day.

Meghan C. Stiffler

To my Mom and Dad—thanks for always being on my team.

Bridget V. Dever

Foreword by Series Editor

Meeting the Training Need

The gap between science and practice in child mental health service delivery is huge and well documented (O'Connell et al. 2009). To fill this gap, better training of education personnel, such as teachers, school counselors, special educators, school psychologists, school social workers, school administrators, etc., is required. This gap in the educational system must be filled in particular, as schools are increasingly being recognized as the most promising institution for mental health service delivery. Universal mental health screening has been prioritized for implementation by legislation and regulation governing schools in Arkansas, Connecticut, Georgia, Indiana, Louisiana, Minnesota, Oregon, Texas, Utah, Washington, Minnesota, Nebraska, Nevada, and Virginia (NAMI 2013).

These legislative initiatives are rooted in compelling data documenting the need for better services. For example, the first comprehensive children's mental health surveillance report by the Centers for Disease Control and Prevention (CDC 2013) concluded that:

- One in five children suffer from a mental health disorder in any given year.
- Suicide was the second leading cause of death in children between 12 and 17 years of age in 2010.
- The prevalence rate of mental health disorders *increases* with child age.
- The cost to American society of these disorders was estimated at $247 billion per year

But what about children who have never been referred, diagnosed, or deemed eligible for special education or related services at school or in their community? How do we identify and serve children with risk; those children who are pre-depressive, mildly anxious, or more active and inattentive than normal but do not meet the diagnostic criteria, those who have been called *subsyndromal* (Cantwell 1996)? Employing a health care metaphor, these might be children who are "pre-hypertensive" or "pre-diabetic." On the other hand, youth in the health care system are identified with such risk through routine, typically annual, screening via urinalysis, blood pressure checks, etc. This universal screening of all children for health risk, however, does not have a counterpart in the behavioral, emotional, or social domains. Thus, we do not routinely detect mental health risk among children and take steps to reduce this risk.

Failure to identify youth with risk sets the stage for risk to become disorder or disability. Youth with subsyndromal problems often have the same impairment in daily living as those who meet diagnostic criteria. In the case of adolescent depression, for example, a review of 27 studies found that children with subsyndromal symptoms suffered from significant impairments both inside and outside of school (Bertha and Balázs 2013). The results were similar for an analogous review of 18 studies of children with subsyndromal problems associated with attention deficit hyperactivity disorder (ADHD; Balázs and Keresztény 2014). These data provide weight to the evidence that universal screening is needed as the first step to engaging in prevention practices. In fact, considerable research indicates that in the absence of valid universal screening both under- (Forness et al. 1998) and overidentification of children with mental health risk abound (particularly for boys of color; Gregory et al. 2010).

Universal mental health risk screening may not be implemented for a variety of reasons including funding, staffing, or lack of policy mandate. There is, however, another root cause of this failure to deploy valid methods of detection and associated preventive interventions—professional knowledge and skill deficits. In higher education in both the USA and elsewhere, the existence of coursework serves as an indication of the degree to which a topic is valued during training. How many undergraduate and graduate courses on universal mental health screening are currently available? At the time of this writing I found a single course. This lack of training, and subsequent skill deficit, particularly among education personnel, has also long been recognized. In this regard, O'Connell et al. (2009) observed:

> Neither the core curriculum for a bachelor's degree nor the process for obtaining a teaching certificate anticipate that teachers will be prepared to recognize risk factors or detect early evidence of MEB [mental, emotional, or behavioral] disorders in their pupils. Coursework for education degree students includes descriptions of mental disorders (along with physical disorders and retardation), but it does not systematically include how to identify, intervene, or refer children at risk for MEB disorders (pp. 366–367).

We need this book because it provides a lucid and authoritative treatise of a topic that serves as the necessary but insufficient first step in the process of implementing comprehensive prevention service delivery for mental health problems in schools. I am grateful to Drs. Stiffler and Dever for sharing their expertise, and am hopeful that trainers of educational personnel will use their expertise included herein to widen the scope of their practice training.

Randy W. Kamphaus
University of Oregon

References

Balázs, J., & Keresztény, Á. (2014). Subthreshold attention deficit hyperactivity in children and adolescents: A systematic review. *European Child & Adolescent Psychiatry, 23*(6), 393–408.
Bertha, E. A., & Balázs, J. (2013). Subthreshold depression in adolescence: A systematic review. *European Child & Adolescent Psychiatry, 22*(10), 589–603.
Cantwell, D.P. (1996). Classification of child and adolescent psychopathology. *Journal of Child Psychology and Psychiatry, 37,* 3–12.
Centers for Disease Control and Prevention (2013). Mental health surveillance among children—United States, 2005–2011. *Morbidity and Mortality Weekly Report Supplement, 62*(2), 1–35.
Forness, S. R., Cluett, S. E., Ramey, C. T., Ramey, S. L., Zima, B. T., Hsu, C. et al. (1998). Special education identification of head start children with emotional and behavioral disorders in second grade. *Journal of Emotional and Behavioral Disorders, 6*(4), 194–204.
Gregory, A., Skiba, R. J., & Noguera, P. A. (2010). The achievement pap and the discipline gap: Two sides of the same coin? *Educational Researcher, 39*(1), 59–68.
National Alliance on Mental Illness. (2013). State legislation report: Trends, themes, and best practices in state mental health legislation. http://www2.nami.org/Content/NavigationMenu/State_Advocacy/Tools_for_Leaders/2013StateLegislationReportFinal.pdf.
O'Connell, M. E., Boat, T., & Warner, K. E. (2009). *Preventing mental, emotional, and behavioral disorders among young people: Progress and possibilities.* Washington, D.C.: National Academies Press.

Acknowledgments

This book would never have been possible without the contributions of many individuals, and we are so grateful for their collaboration in different stages of this project.

We are most appreciative of the support from Randy Kamphaus, the editor of this series. This volume became a reality due to his guidance, encouragement, and mentorship throughout the entire process.

To all the students and colleagues who provided suggestions for revisions, additions, and subtractions, your feedback was instrumental in framing this book for a broader audience of readers. Thank you for your willingness to read our words, sometimes multiple times, to help us get them right.

Finally, it is important to acknowledge the school districts, administrators, school psychologists, school counselors, teachers, and students who have contributed much of the practical wisdom that served as inspiration for this book. It is only through those collaborations that we can continue to work toward achieving our goal of supporting the mental health needs of children and adolescents.

Meghan C. Stiffler
Bridget V. Dever

Contents

About the Authors

Meghan C. Stiffler, Ph.D., is currently a licensed psychologist in Texas. She has received numerous recognitions for her academic accomplishments. She was awarded the prestigious Presidential Fellowship to obtain her doctoral degree in educational psychology at the University of Georgia, where she conducted 4 years of research, with Professor Randy W. Kamphaus, on school-based mental health screening. She has quickly become a recognized expert on this topic because of her journal articles and many presentations on screening issues, such as the use of multiple informants and multiple gates in universal screening programs. She previously worked as a school psychologist with Cypress Fairbanks Independent School District in Houston, Texas, for 3 years.

Bridget V. Dever, Ph.D., is an assistant professor of school psychology at Lehigh University. Dr. Dever graduated from the University of Michigan in 2009 with a Ph.D. from the Combined Program in Education and Psychology. Her research interests include behavioral, emotional, and academic risk, promoting educational resilience, and achievement motivation among at-risk students. Her work includes peer-reviewed publications in *Journal of School Psychology, Psychological Assessment, Journal of Psychoeducational Assessment, Contemporary Educational Psychology, Prevention Science, and School Psychology Quarterly,* several book chapters, and over 50 scholarly presentations. Dr. Dever has expertise in universal screening data collection, management, analysis, and synthesis, because of her involvement in several large-scale school-based research programs, including the coordination of a 3-year universal screening program that included more than 8000 students.

About the Authors

Chapter 1
Introduction

The Motivation for This Volume

Although this volume is, of course, motivated by decades of research and practice, the true motivating force for this book is the children in our schools who suffer from or are at risk for behavioral and emotional difficulties. As stated in Dr. Kamphaus' foreword, it is critical to amass what we know, and what we *do not* know, about mental health screening in the schools to better train our practitioners, researchers, and administrators concerning the detection of mental health risk. This volume is informed by seminal work in the field, emerging research findings, and our own applied experiences with screening in the schools. We hope that it will not only help with training teachers, school psychologists, and others with an interest in the topic but will also serve to inspire our fellow colleagues to continue to work toward a model of universal screening for mental health risk in the schools.

As others have noted (e.g., Bruhn et al. 2014), tragedies such as the shootings at Columbine High School, Sandy Hook Elementary School, and others have sparked increased dialogue about the issue of mental health in our schools. In fact, when we have identified our interest in mental health screening to others in the past, we are often asked whether we are trying to identify school shooters through screening. The answer is no, but that is not intended to be a disappointing answer, as we feel the question is somewhat ill-conceived. Just as modern medicine does not aim to detect a rare and unlikely heart condition moments before it takes hold, our work is not designed to detect the statistically rare and monumentally devastating incidence of a school shooting immediately prior to its occurrence. Instead, mental health screening is intended as a prevention tool to detect risk for disorder *before* a diagnosis is made, *before* symptoms become increasingly severe, and hopefully long before that risk escalates to tragedy.

In the wake of the Sandy Hook Elementary School shooting, the Council for Children with Behavioral Disorders issued a statement (CCBD 2012), which included the goals of screening for mental health risk and training practitioners about mental health issues. In addition, the 2004 reauthorization of the Individuals with Disabilities Education Act (IDEA) indicated that schools may elect to use up to

M. C. Stiffler, B. V. Dever, *Mental Health Screening at School*, Contemporary Issues in Psychological Assessment, DOI 10.1007/978-3-319-19171-3_1

15 % of their IDEA funds toward efforts to identify and intervene with students at-risk for academic or behavioral/emotional problems (IDEA 2004). Despite these efforts, it is approximated that 12–13 % of the schools screen for mental health risk (Bruhn et al. 2014). The good news is that this figure has increased since 2005, when Romer and McIntosh reported that mental health screening occurred in about 2 % of schools. However, it is clear that we have a long way to go before universal screening in all schools becomes a reality.

We do not believe that the lack of universal screening for mental health in schools is due to any lack of interest or concern on the part of administrators, school psychologists, teachers, parents, and other stakeholders. Instead, we acknowledge that the reality for those individuals includes long days filled with trying to meet the academic, social, emotional, and physical needs of our nation's youth. Increased research and increased awareness are not enough to institute practical changes; instead, there must be a pipeline of information from the researchers, from those who do this work in the schools, back to the practitioners who would be able to learn from our work (and our mistakes). We hope that this volume will be a starting point for getting this valuable information into the hands of those who might be able to use it for prevention and early intervention in the schools.

Organization for This Volume

With so many choices in terms of screening instruments, informants, procedures, etc., it is no wonder that more schools do not screen universally for mental health risk. The accumulation of knowledge in the field is such a valuable place to start, but is often difficult for practitioners to both locate and navigate. We hope that this volume will begin to answer some of the questions regarding the "Who, what, when, where, why, and how?" of screening for mental health risk in schools.

Chapter 2 provides the reader with a presentation of the history of screening practices, starting with screening in the medical field. To understand mental health screening, it is critical to understand the theory behind screening and early detection more broadly. This chapter also includes information on the history of mental health assessment and classification in the USA, to frame our later discussion more broadly in a historical context that is grounded both in medicine and psychology. This chapter provides a comprehensive review of the "what" and "why" that resulted in mental health screening more broadly.

In Chapter 3, we focus more on the "where," with a discussion of current systems of identification. While we start with information on mental health screening in more clinical settings, this chapter presents the argument for the need for mental health screening in schools more specifically. The school remains the focal context throughout the remainder of the book, as schools provide a unique opportunity to conduct what could be truly universal screening among all school-aged children.

Chapters 4 through 6 are the chapters what will likely be of most interest to those who want to better understand the current "toolkit" of available screening procedures. Collectively, these chapters cover the "Who, when, and how?" of mental health screening. First, Chapter 4 provides information concerning broadband and specific screening instruments that are available for use. Although we attempted to include as many instruments as possible, the nascent field of mental health screening in schools is constantly evolving. Therefore, while every effort was made to include those that are the most widely used and empirically based, it is critical to continue to compile information regarding such instruments in a way that is accessible to practitioners.

Chapter 5 situates mental health screening within a response to intervention (RtI) framework, as this is often an area of emphasis in current training models. Here we review the RtI model and discuss universal screening as a Tier I effort to inform prevention and intervention. We believe that the RtI framework is a useful way to conceptualize the integration of universal screening, early intervention, and regular progress monitoring within a school- or district-wide system of service delivery.

Chapter 6 provides the reader with an overview of the multiple-gating approach to screening and service delivery. As multiple informants often participate in this approach, information regarding the selection of informants for screening and assessment is also included in this chapter. Finally, an example of a widely used multiple-gate system is presented here as well.

In Chapter 7, we transition to applied examples of our own screening work in the schools. In this chapter, we convey how our screening program was based on both research evidence and practical decisions. These examples are not meant to serve as an ultimate blueprint for screening; rather, they are presented as concrete examples regarding both the benefits and challenges of conducting universal screening in schools.

Finally, Chapter 8 summarizes some of the current issues and future directions in mental health screening. Although this volume introduces the reader to accumulating research in the field, the more we read and the more we do, the more clear it becomes that there is so much more for us to study, know, and understand. The budding researcher may find this chapter particularly helpful when attempting to decide, "What next?" concerning future scholarship that is needed in the field.

Conclusion

In summary, we truly hope this volume serves to generate and sustain conversations about the need for and implementation of mental health screening in schools. Without proper guidance and support, practitioners in our schools might see universal screening as a noble but insurmountable goal. This book is meant to make the goal of universal screening more concrete and attainable. Trainers, researchers, teachers, school psychologists, administrators, and other stakeholders will likely find different pieces of this book useful to guide their future screening work. As emerging scholars ourselves, we welcome continued dialogue about the importance and implementation of mental health screening in schools, so that we can better serve our true audience of interest—our students, our children, and our youth.

References

Bruhn, A. L., Woods-Groves, S., & Huddle, S. (2014). A preliminary investigation of emotional and behavioral screening practices in K-12 schools. *Education and Treatment of Children, 37,* 611–634.

Council for Children with Behavioral Disorders (2012). Response to Sandy Hook tragedy. http://cecblog.typepad.com/files/ccbd-response-to-sandy-hook-tragedy-w-signatures.pdf. Accessed 31 March 2015.

Individuals with Disabilities Education Improvement Act, 20 U.S.C. § 1400 (2004).

Romer, D., & McIntosh, M. (2005). The roles and perspectives of school mental health professionals in promoting adolescent mental health. In D. L. Evans, E. B. Foa, R. E. Gur, H. Hendin, C. P. O'Brien, M. E. P. Seligman, & B. T. Walsh (Eds.), *Treating and preventing adolescent mental health disorders: What we know and what we don't know* (pp. 598–615). New York: Oxford University Press.

Chapter 2
History of Screening Practices, Mental Health Assessment, and Classification in the USA

General Principles of Screening

In 1951, the Commission on Chronic Illness Conference on Preventive Aspects of Chronic Disease defined screening as "the presumptive identification of unrecognized disease or defect by the application of tests, examinations, or other procedures which can be applied rapidly. Screening tests sort out apparently well persons who probably have a disease from those who probably do not. A screening test is not intended to be diagnostic. Persons with positive or suspicious findings must be referred to their physicians for diagnosis and necessary treatment" (Wilson and Jungner 1968, p. 11). Wilson and Jungner explained that "early detection aims at discovering and curing conditions which have already produced pathological change but which have not so far reached a stage at which medical aid is sought spontaneously." Thus, the objective of medical screening is not to diagnose, but to identify possible problems earlier than would naturally occur so as to increase the probability of curing the condition through early treatment and intervention.

A second purpose of screening, especially in less developed countries, is to control the spread of communicable diseases. According to Morabia and Zhang (2004), screening programs became possible when four conditions were met: the availability of simple, valid, and acceptable forms of screening tests; the discovery of effective treatments; the establishment of a theory of screening; and wide access to health care. The importance of the development of valid screening instruments as well as proven effective treatments prior to implementing a screening program cannot be overemphasized (Moyer et al. 2008). Screening is only worth the effort if early detection and treatment leads to better outcomes than would be expected without earlier detection.

In 1968, the World Health Organization (WHO; Wilson and Jungner 1968) provided guidelines for effective health screening:

1. The condition should be an important health problem that carries with it notable morbidity and mortality.
2. There should be an accepted treatment for patients with recognized disease.
3. Facilities for diagnosis and treatment should be available.

M. C. Stiffler, B. V. Dever, *Mental Health Screening at School*, Contemporary Issues in Psychological Assessment, DOI 10.1007/978-3-319-19171-3_2

4. There should be a recognizable latent or early symptomatic stage.
5. There should be a suitable test or examination.
6. The test should be acceptable to the population.
7. The natural history of the condition, including development from latent to declared disease, should be adequately understood.
8. There should be an agreed policy on whom to treat as patients.
9. The cost of finding, diagnosing, and treating patients should be economically balanced in relation to the anticipated overall expenditure on medical care.
10. Case-finding should be a continuing process and not a "once and for all" project.

These guidelines have served to frame the process of mental health screening. Generally, it appears that mental health disorders meet the criteria that would facilitate screening. Mental health disorders are important health problems with known morbidity, mortality, and costs to society (Campaign for Mental Health Reform 2005; United States Public Health Service 2000). Evidence-based medications as well as psychosocial interventions exist that have been found to effectively treat most mental health disorders (New Freedom Commission on Mental Health 2003). A number of effective or promising treatments exist for many mental disorders in children, including cognitive behavioral therapy and selective serotonin reuptake inhibitors for depression (Kaslow and Thompson 1998), parent training and multisystemic therapy for conduct disorder (Brestan and Eyberg 1998), and psychostimulants and behavioral training of teachers for attention-deficit/hyperactivity disorder (ADHD; Pelham et al. 1998). Research has also shown that identifying and treating children early, before their emotional and behavioral problems are diagnosable, can minimize the long-term detriment of mental disorders as well as reduce overall health-care burden and costs (Aos et al. 2004; Campaign for Mental Health Reform 2005). Evidence supporting the use of screening programs with mental health disorders is presented throughout this text; however, it is clear that based on the information provided thus far mental health disorders far surpass the minimum criteria necessary for screening programs to potentially succeed in facilitating early intervention and prevention efforts.

History of Screening Practices in the USA

Screening in the Army

The history of screening practices in the USA can be traced back to psychological roots in the late nineteenth and early twentieth centuries. One of the oldest screening programs recorded was employed by the Division of Psychology within the Medical Department of the US Army during World War I. In 1917, the army began administering mental tests to officers, new conscripts, and enlisted men "to help to eliminate from the army at the earliest possible moment those recruits whose defective intelligence would make them a menace to the military organization" (from Morabia and Zhang, p. 464). Those whose test results indicated that they were at risk for difficulties were referred for more detailed individual psychological examinations. In 1918, Robert Woodworth published the Woodworth Personal Data Sheet (Woodworth 1918) as part of a national effort to screen potential soldiers for psychiatric disorders before allowing them into the US Army. This instrument allowed for the screening of large numbers of recruits quickly without the need for trained interviewers (Kleinmuntz 1967).

During World War II, a standardized paper-and-pencil test, later named the neuropsychiatric screening adjunct (NSA) test, was developed by the Research Branch for the Surgeon General in order to identify individuals with psychiatric disorders and eliminate them from military services. The army had planned on evaluating the theory behind the screening test as well as the economics and practical issues involved in implementing the screening program. However, because the NSA test was officially adopted for use just a few months before the end of the war it was not utilized enough to allow for the evaluation of its impact (Morabia and Zhang 2004).

Presently, the US Veterans Administration (VA) continues to implement mental health screening programs. Because of the high rates of psychiatric disorders found following the Vietnam and Persian Gulf Wars as well as the failure of predeployment screenings to reduce the incidence of psychological problems, the focus of screening over the past 10 years has shifted from predeployment screening to the detection of mental health problems following deployment. In June 2004, the VA issued a national directive to initiate the Afghan and Iraq Post-Deployment Screen, consisting of brief, previously validated instruments used to detect symptoms of posttraumatic stress disorder (PTSD), depression, and high-risk alcohol use among veterans who seek VA healthcare (Seal et al. 2008). However, more recent initiatives have focused on screening for mental health concerns earlier in the process, during the recruitment phase. For example, in May 2014, the House of Representatives passed a bill requiring the National Institutes of Health to design a universal screening instrument for mental health issues among recruits, which would replace the largely informal system for detecting preexisting concerns that is currently in place.

Newborn Screening

In the 1960s, the first large-scale, state-mandated newborn screening program was implemented to identify the presence of a genetic metabolic disorder called Phenylketonuria (PKU). PKU is an autosomal recessive genetic disorder characterized by a deficiency in the enzyme phenylalanine hydroxylase (PAH), which is necessary to metabolize the amino acid phenylalanine to the amino acid tyrosine. If left untreated, PKU can cause problems with brain development, leading to progressive mental retardation and seizures. Though there is no cure for PKU, by screening all infants at birth before the disorder manifests any observable symptoms, and placing those who test positive on a diet low in phenylalanine and high in tyrosine, it is possible to prevent the irreversible effects of the condition.

As new screening techniques have developed and individual disease genes have been identified, states have added a range of other conditions to their mandated newborn screening programs and the development of pilot screening programs has begun for numerous genetic and prenatal conditions including Down's syndrome, neural tube defects, Tay–Sachs disease, and cystic fibrosis. In 2005, a report released by the American College of Medical Genetics (ACMG) called for all states to adopt a core newborn screening panel consisting of 29 primary disorders as well as 25 secondary disorders (Watson et al. 2006).

Some researchers have voiced concern over the rapid expansion of recommended newborn screenings, stating that "a new condition should be added to the mandatory panel only when there is an established screening test and good evidence that the condition causes serious harm and that the harm can be avoided if the infant is diagnosed and treated immediately after birth" (Baily and Murray 2008, p. 25). PKU is an excellent example of a mandatory, universal screening program that can be justified under these criteria as well as the criteria provided by Wilson and Jungner (1968). However, Moyer et al. (2008, p. 36) feel that "the push for expanded newborn screening has bypassed traditional, evidence-based decision-making processes at both the state and federal level." They argue that many of the disorders identified by the ACMG are not yet fully understood, have no proven treatment, or have treatments that are helpful only after clinical presentation, and should therefore not be on the mandatory screening panel as we should not mandate screening for a condition simply because we have the technology to do so. Some parents may not want to be informed that their child has the condition if there is no medical treatment or benefit to early detection. Other factors that must be considered include the natural history and progression of the disorder, the cost-effectiveness of the screening, the benefit–harm ratio of conducting the screening (e.g., will screening lead to unnecessary worry and labeling?), the effectiveness versus the risks of treatments and preventative strategies, the validity of the screening instrument, and the state's ability to create and sustain a system that works for each disorder. Many of these issues also pertain to the issue of universal mental health screening and are discussed later in the text.

Medical Screening

In 1957, the commission on chronic disease indicated that screening might be effective for the following medical conditions: pulmonary tuberculosis, visual defects (including chronic glaucoma), hearing defects, syphilis, diabetes, hypertensive disease, and cancers of the skin, mouth, breast, cervix, and rectum (Wilson and Jungner 1968). Currently, screening for many of these conditions is conducted by physicians (e.g., cancers, hypertensive disease) or at schools (hearing, vision). However, screening for some diseases is no longer relevant due to the success of previous screening programs in eliminating these conditions from the population (e.g., tuberculosis, syphilis).

Syphilis

Following World War II, syphilis screening increased significantly due to the simultaneous availability of a rapid test and a quick and effective treatment. In June 1944, penicillin became available to the US Public Health Service and was made available for treating syphilis in the civilian population (Morabia and Zhang 2004). Additionally, two syphilis screening tests became available: non-treponemal tests and treponemal antibody tests. Both types of syphilis screening tests were found to suffer from low sensitivity or the proportion of actual positives which are correctly identified as such (ranging from 0.78 to 0.86), but had excellent specificity or the proportion of negatives which are correctly identified as such (>0.97; Larsen et al. 1995). Because of the technical difficulty and costliness of administering the treponemal antibody tests, non-treponemal tests were used for screening and treponemal tests for secondary confirmation. At the end of World War II, of the 15 million men who entered the armed services, 750,000 screened positively for syphilis. In the 1950s and 1960s, a number of screening "blitzes" were performed, consisting of a large-scale examination and treatment of all identified contacts of patients with syphilis (Morabia and Zhang 2004). By the mid-1950s, reported cases of syphilis had declined so sharply that mass testing was eliminated and replaced with selective testing of suspected high-risk subgroups. Since the 1960s, routine serological screening programs have been discontinued in many states (Johnson and Farnie 1994). Overall, the historical effectiveness of syphilis screening provides an example of the long-term public health benefits and cost-effectiveness of a well-executed screening program.

Diabetes Mellitus

Around 1946, following the discovery of insulin in 1923 and an increase in deaths from diabetes, one of the first large-scale community diabetes screenings was completed in Oxford, Massachusetts by the US Public Health Services. Approximately 70.6% of the 4983 residents received both urine and blood glucose testing, and the prevalence of diabetes was found to be 1.7%. Evidence also exists that glucose screening in specific groups was performed prior to this, including army screening in an attempt to eliminate those with diabetes from military service during World War I (Morabia and Zhang 2004).

Several types of tests have been utilized in screening for diabetes. The urinary glucose test has been found to have low sensitivity, and was therefore used only when blood testing was not available or too expensive. Blood glucose screening (including random blood glucose tests and fasting whole blood glucose tests) was found to have higher sensitivity and specificity and was often used along with a urinary test to maximize sensitivity. The oral glucose tolerance test (OGTT) was later developed, but was only used when other tests were inadequate due to inconvenience of administration (Harting and Glenn 1951).

Currently, diabetes screening is recommended for many people at certain stages of life and with certain risk factors. Many health-care providers recommend universal screening for adults at age 40 or 50, and often periodically thereafter. Earlier screening is typically recommended for those with risk factors such as obesity, family history of diabetes, or membership in a high-risk ethnicity group (Hispanic, Native American, Afro-Caribbean, Pacific Island, and South Asian ancestry; Lee et al. 2007). Recently, the United States Preventive Services Task Force (2008, p. 846) recommended that all asymptomatic adults with sustained blood pressure (either treated or untreated) greater than 135/80 mm Hg be screened for type 2 diabetes based upon "evidence that early treatment prevents long-term adverse outcomes including cardiovascular events, visual impairment, renal failure, and amputation." The screening test varies according to circumstances and local policy, and may include a random or fasting blood glucose test, a blood glucose test 2 h after 75 g of glucose, or an oral glucose tolerance test.

Cancer

Currently, mass screenings for numerous cancers (including cervical, breast, and prostate) are implemented on a routine basis. Before World War II, only pilot programs of cancer detection had been conducted. Following the development of the cervical cancer cytological test (e.g., Pap smear) by Papanicolaou and Traut in 1943, cervical cancer screenings were successfully conducted on a wide scale. Cervical cancer is an excellent candidate for screening as it is detectable in the preclinical phase, thus increasing chances of cure and improved prognosis. Although subject to error at several levels, the Pap smear has been found to have sensitivities ranging from 0.89 to 1.0 (Patten 1969 from Morabia and Zhang 2004). Studies have found that since the widespread use of the Pap smear in the 1970s, the incidence and death rates from cervical cancer in the USA have dropped almost 50 %. Despite this decrease, cervical cancer continues to be the second most common cancer among women (Catranis 2005).

In 2003, the American College of Obstetricians and Gynecologists (ACOG) issued new, evidence-based practice guidelines regarding Pap smear frequency stating that as some women need more frequent screening, an increasing number of women no longer need annual cervical cancer screening. They cautioned that annual pelvic examinations are still advised for all women over age 21. Generally, ACOG now recommends an initial Pap test approximately 3 years after the first sexual intercourse experience or by age 21, whichever comes first. Women up to age 30 should continue to undergo annual Pap testing whereas those over age 30 can undergo screening less frequently; the ACOG states that if a woman age 30 or older has negative results on three consecutive annual Pap smears, she may then have her repeat Pap smears every 2–3 years (Catranis 2005).

Mass breast cancer screening began in the 1960s following the development of the mammogram as a screening instrument. The efficacy of breast cancer screening has been demonstrated in randomized controlled trials (RCTs) and observational studies; thus, most organizations that issue recommendations endorse regular mammography as an important part of preventive care (Smith et al. 2003). In 2003, the American Cancer Society updated their recommendations regarding breast cancer screening to suggest that women of average risk begin having annual mammograms at age 40. They also indicated that women at increased risk of breast cancer might benefit from additional screening strategies such as earlier initiation of annual screening, shorter screening intervals, or the addition of screening modalities other than mammography and physical examination such as ultrasound or magnetic resonance imaging. However, the American Cancer Society concluded that the evidence was insufficient to justify recommendations for any of these alternative screening approaches (Smith et al. 2003).

As one can see, the USA has a rich history of screening practices that continue to be implemented today. The principles of prevention, early detection, and universal care were first applied to the field of infectious disease through the use of mass screenings, early treatment, and prevention strategies including vaccinations, water safety, and other public hygiene practices. Infants are screened for a number of genetic diseases at birth, and children are routinely screened for hearing, vision, and scoliosis at school and pediatrician visits. Universal screening approaches are now standard practice for many health concerns and have been largely successful in minimizing the negative effects and, in some cases, eliminating particular diseases from the population. Despite the widespread implementation of screening for medical concerns, screening for mental health issues unfortunately has lagged behind.

Mental Health Assessment and Classification

History of Mental Health Assessment

Experimental psychology can trace its roots back to the opening of Wilhelm Wundt's experimental psychology lab in Germany in 1879. Wundt and his assistant, Cattell, found individual differences on measures of sensory abilities and reaction time. These types of measures were incorporated into intelligence tests developed by Cattell and Sir Francis Galton. Galton believed that intelligence was inherited and could be objectively measured, and developed a battery of tests that he thought would allow him to study the inheritance of intelligence. In addition to intelligence, Galton was also intrigued by the measurement of "character," citing a personality inventory developed by Benjamin Franklin in order to demonstrate the utility of personality measurement (Kamphaus and Frick 2002). Therefore, formal psychological assessment stemmed from other efforts to measure individual differences.

Additionally, the psychological testing of soldiers in the US Army during World War I and the development of the previously mentioned Woodworth Personal Data Sheet (Woodworth 1918) can be considered two of the main impetuses for the development of more formal and widely used measures of psychological functioning.

The Woodworth Personal Data Sheet, consisting of 116 questions about daydreaming, worry, mood, and other problems, has been described as "the linear ancestor of all subsequent personality inventories, schedules, and questionnaires" (DuBois 1970, p. 94). French and Hale (1990) suggest that the Woodworth Personal Data Sheet served as the foundation for future scales such as the Thurstone Personality Scale and the Allport Ascendance-Submission Scale, among others. The success of World War I applications of psychological testing demonstrated the practical value of psychology to society.

As reviewed in a previous section, following World War II the US VA began using psychologists in large numbers to diagnose and treat returning veterans suffering from significant psychological problems such as PTSD. Psychologists began developing new methods for assessing personality and psychological functioning to meet this need. Since this time, the assessment of personality, behavior, emotions, and social functioning has increased dramatically and expanded into a wide variety of areas including education, counseling, personnel selection, and even online dating services.

In the early half of the twentieth century, projective assessment techniques were the most popular forms of psychological assessment (Kamphaus and Frick 2002). Projective techniques were based upon the idea that the use of ambiguous stimuli would encourage individuals to reveal information that they otherwise would not share when questioned directly (Chandler 1990). Examples of popular projective techniques include the thematic apperception test (TAT), the Rorschach test, sentence completion tasks, and drawing tasks such as house-tree-person or the Kinetic Family Drawing. These techniques continue to be used regularly, although it may be argued that objective techniques are more popular today.

Objective techniques are considered to be more empirically based than the projective techniques described above. Empirical methods and psychometric science have typically been used to develop these measures as well as to interpret their results. The Minnesota Multiphasic Personality Inventory (MMPI; Hathaway and McKinney 1942) was one of the first tests to use an empirical approach to personality test development. Rather than depending on the test authors' theory of personality for item selection *(rational-theoretical approach)*, as was most popular at that time, the MMPI used an item-selection method called *empirical criterion keying* (Martin 1988). Generally, this technique involves selecting items that routinely differentiate clinical groups from samples of controls, and further distinguish clinical groups from each other, without taking the content of the items into account. In the 1950s, the personality inventory for children (PIC), an offshoot of the MMPI, was developed using factor-analytic methods for the personality assessment of children.

Personality Versus Behavioral Assessment

Historically, personality assessment focused on identifying the more enduring and stable characteristics or traits of a person and his or her pattern of interaction with the environment. The most popular examples of this type of classification would be the MMPI described above as well as the big five personality traits or factors discovered by Tupes and Christal (1961) through multiple analyses of numerous data sets from scales of bipolar personality descriptors (Kamphaus and Frick 2002). These five factors are: introversion/extroversion, agreeableness, conscientiousness, emotional stability, and culture, intellect, openness and are assessed by having the individual complete a forced-choice item format questionnaire in which adjectives are used as personality descriptors.

During the rise of popularity of behaviorism, psychologists began focusing on smaller, observable units of analysis or "behaviors" rather than the trait-based methods described above. As described by Martin (1988, p. 13), "Behavior is differentiated from traits or dispositions because the latter may only be seen if behavior is aggregated over relatively long periods of time and in a number of environmental contexts. Classical examples of observed behaviors of interest to child psychologists include tantrum behavior among young children, aggressive interactions with peers, attempts at conversation initiation, and so forth." In this way, an emphasis is placed on the way an individual behaves, adjusts, or reacts to environmental stimuli. Kamphaus and Frick (2002, p. 3) have presented three "distinguishing features of behavioral assessment methods." First, behavioral assessment has a different theoretical foundation than trait-based psychological assessment; behavioral assessment draws heavily on behavioral theories such as Skinner's operant conditioning and is often considered more empirically based. Second, unlike the medical model of assessment, which assumes that symptoms are caused by underlying medical conditions which must be measured, diagnosed, and treated in order to eliminate the symptoms, behavioral assessment emphasizes the measurement and treatment of the behaviors or symptoms themselves. Lastly, behavioral assessment places greater emphasis on the assessment of discrete behaviors.

More recently, the use of rating scales for the assessment of child psychopathology has become increasingly popular and widespread. Several behavior rating scales such as those developed by Achenbach, Conners, Reynolds, and Kamphaus have begun to blur the line between behavioral and trait-based assessment through the assessment of dimensions of behavior such as internalizing and externalizing behaviors (Kamphaus and Frick 2002). Internalizing problems are often described as "overcontrolled" adjustment difficulties such as problems with anxiety, inhibition, depression, somatic complaints, and social withdrawal. Children with externalizing problems, on the other hand, may be described as "undercontrolled" and have difficulties with aggression, hyperactivity, conduct problems, and acting-out behavior (Edelbrock 1979). These two dimensions of child psychopathology have been supported by many factor-analytic investigations of both parent and teacher rating scales as well as by concurrent validity studies (Edelbrock 1979). The robust evidence of the existence of the internalizing and externalizing dimensions has led to their use in the development of many child rating scales including the Achenbach Child Behavior Checklist (CBCL; Achenbach 1991) and the Behavior Assessment System for Children (BASC and BASC-2; Reynolds and Kamphaus 1992, 2004). More information about these and similar instruments is presented in Chapter 4.

Why Classify?

Classification is a natural human activity that helps us make sense of our world. We are constantly grouping people and things we encounter based upon similarities and differences so as to organize and understand these things more efficiently. People informally assess and classify personality and behavior every day. Mothers and teachers describe children as sensitive, difficult, inattentive, or easygoing. Upon meeting someone, we quickly assess and classify him or her as someone we would like to get to know better or someone we would rather avoid in the future.

One of the primary purposes of mental health assessment is to classify or diagnose individuals so as to make decisions regarding appropriate courses of treatment or intervention. *Classification* can be broadly defined as the systematic arranging or distributing of phenomena into groups or categories according to established criteria or sets of rules. In psychological assessment, two levels of classification might be delineated: (1) to determine when psychological functioning is abnormal, deviant, or in need of treatment; and (2) to determine the specific types of psychopathology that are present (Kamphaus and Frick 2002). *Diagnosis* may be considered a specialized, more restrictive form of classification focused on the categorization of diseases and consistent with the second type of classification described above. Mental health screening, on the other hand, focuses on the first level of classification in which we determine whether an individual is generally at-risk for or exhibiting subsyndromal mental health symptoms requiring intervention rather than officially diagnosing and differentiating between disorders (Dever and Kamphaus 2013).

The classification of mental disorders can be traced back to the earliest times in recorded history. Greek writings referred to four terms, "melancholia," "hysteria," "mania," and "paranoia," which are still used today (Blashfield 1998). During the middle ages, mental disorders were considered a sign of the presence of something evil, and were therefore under the domain of religious authorities rather than physicians or scientists. Then, around the late 1700s, records suggest a shift in this way of thinking as, for example, King George III of England was treated for his psychosis by medical personnel rather than religious authorities. An increasing interest in psychopathology during the nineteenth century led to the development of several mental disorder classification systems.

William A. Hammond, a nineteenth century neurologist with an interest in psychiatry, argued for six possible principles around which one could organize a classification system:

1. Anatomical organization by the part of the brain that is affected.
2. Physiological organization by the physiological system in the brain.
3. Etiological organization by supposed causes.
4. Psychological organization based upon a functional view of the mind.
5. Pathological organization by observable, morbid alterations in the brain.
6. Clinical organization based upon descriptive clusters of symptoms.

Hammond indicated that the anatomical, physiological, and etiological principles were optimal for the design of a classification system, but that they could not be used at that time due to insufficient science (Blashfield 1998). Therefore, he utilized the psychological principle to create his classification system indicating six major categories of mental disorders:

1. Perceptual insanities (e.g., hallucinations)
2. Intellectual insanities (e.g., delusional thoughts)
3. Emotional insanities (e.g., melancholia or depression)
4. Volitional insanities (e.g., abulomania)
5. Compound insanities (i.e., disorders affecting more than one area of the mind, comorbidity)
6. Constitutional insanities (i.e., disorders with specific causes such as choreic insanity) (Blashfield 1998).

Around the turn of the century, a German psychiatrist named Emil Kraepelin was the medical director at an insane asylum in eastern Prussia. While there, he published a number of psychology studies and textbooks about psychopathology organized around what he believed to be the major categories of mental disorders (Kraepelin 1902/1896). As opposed to Sigmund Freud, Kraepelin argued that psychiatric diseases were mainly caused by biological and genetic disorders. He is credited with classifying what was previously considered to be a unitary concept of psychosis into two distinct forms: manic depression (now seen as comprising a range of mood disorders such as major depression and bipolar disorder), and dementia praecox (or schizophrenia). His fundamental theories on the etiology and diagnosis of psychiatric disorders formed the basis of the major diagnostic systems in use today, including the *American Psychiatric Association's Diagnostic and Statistical Manual* (DSM 1994, 2013) and the World Health Organization's ICD system (Blashfield 1998).

The current classification systems in psychology and psychiatry are riddled with imperfections largely due to the constructs with which these fields must work. Psychological phenomena are inherently messy and do not fit perfectly into categories of normal and abnormal nor into definite, nonoverlapping types of psychopathology. Rather, these constructs tend to fall along dimensions with no clear demarcation of pathology and non-pathology and comorbidity tends to be the rule rather than the exception, especially when dealing with children.

In spite of the challenges in defining psychopathology, most researchers continue to agree that explicit classification is necessary despite its imperfections (Kamphaus and Frick 2002). Blashfield (1998) has described five primary purposes for classification:

1. Creation of a common professional nomenclature.
2. Organization of information.
3. Clinical description.
4. Prediction of outcomes and treatment utility.
5. The development of concepts upon which theories may be based.

Through the development and use of common, operationally defined terminology and classifications, professionals are able to communicate with each other, retrieve information more effectively, predict future behaviors, and document the need for services. Best practice appears to support utilizing our current systems of classification while being aware of and attempting to minimize the dangers and pitfalls of doing so. Two of the main limitations of classification are the information lost through labeling and the illusory break created between normal and pathological psychological functioning when attempting to fit people into clear-cut categories (Kamphaus and Frick 2002).

Categorical Versus Dimensional Models of Classification

Two organizational models of classification often discussed in the literature are the categorical (or medical) model and the dimensional (or multivariate) approach. The *categorical model* assumes a disease entity that differs *qualitatively* from normality, and then defines the symptoms that are indicative of the presence of the disorder. Typically, a sharp distinction is made between disordered and non-disordered individuals. An individual either has the disorder or does not. Optimal methods for assessment using a categorical approach would include structured diagnostic interviews, semistructured or unstructured interviews, collection of historical information, and classroom observations (Kamphaus et al. 2006).

The *dimensional approach*, on the other hand, focuses on *quantitative* distinctions along dimensions of behavior. Empirical methods, usually multivariate statistical procedures including cluster or factor analysis, are used to isolate behavioral dimensions from measures such as behavior rating scales. An individual's level of functioning, across various dimensions of behaviors on a continuum from normal to deviant, is then assessed. Classification is based upon comparing an individual's functioning relative to a representative normative sample (i.e., norm referencing) and designating a certain level of functioning as adequately deviant from the average population as to be significant (Dever and Kamphaus 2013). Methods of assessment would include behavior rating scales completed by multiple informants, formal tests of cognition and achievement, and tests of adaptive behavior (Kamphaus et al. 2006).

Blashfield (1998, pp. 69, 70) outlined a number of tenets of each model (see Table 2.1).

Although these two models are sometimes thought to be competing and mutually exclusive, integrating these models is possible and perhaps ideal as both have their strengths and weaknesses. The relative value and superiority of these two classification models has been frequently debated (Dowdy et al. 2009; Fletcher 1985).

Advantages of the categorical model of classification are quite apparent. By developing clear and concise operationally-defined diagnostic criteria for disorders, diagnostic agreement is increased and communication is improved among professionals for research and treatment development as well as to the public

Table 2.1 Comparison of the categorical and dimensional models of classification

Categorical model	Dimensional model
1. Unit is psychiatric classification of patients	1. Unit is a descriptive variable (e.g., a symptom, characteristic, etc.)
2. Categories should be discrete	2. Dimensions are abstract variables, and represent a continuum
3. The members of a category should be relatively homogeneous	3. The dimensions account for almost as much variance as do the larger number of descriptive variables to which they are related
4. Categories may have some overlap, but this is not intended. Where categories do overlap, the number of patients in these comorbid areas should be relatively small	4. Dimensions may be correlated or independent, but due to relationships among descriptive variables correlations among dimensions are often expected
5. Cluster analytic methods are used to identify categories. Discriminant analysis is used to validate categories	5. Exploratory factor analysis and multidimensional scaling are used to identify dimensions. Confirmatory factor analysis can be used to validate a specific dimensional model

(Dowdy et al. 2009; Kamphaus et al. 2006). The main disadvantages of a categorical system are largely due to the nature of psychopathology itself or, as described by Jablensky (1999), a lack of goodness of fit between our categorical classification system and "clinical reality." Ideally, when using a categorical system, members of given categories or diagnoses should be relatively homogeneous and boundaries between categories should be clear. This does not appear to be the case with current psychological diagnoses as individuals with the same diagnosis are often quite heterogeneous and boundaries between diagnoses are fuzzy. The over-use of atypical disorders, such as those labeled as "Not Otherwise Specified," indicating a failure to meet the set diagnostic criteria, also lead clinicians to question the validity and utility of current diagnostic categories (Kamphaus et al. 2006).

Achenbach and McConaughy (1992) argued that the dichotomous nature of a categorical model fails to account for those children whose problems vary in degree or severity. Research has begun to accumulate suggesting that many child behavior problems such as inattention, hyperactivity, depression, and conduct problems fall along continua in the population (Kamphaus et al. 2006). Due to the continuous, rather than all or none, nature of these behaviors, important information is lost, such as the severity of the disorder (e.g. mild, moderate, or severe) or significant subsyndromal psychopathology that is functionally impairing but below diagnostic thresholds (Hudziak et al. 1999; Scahill et al. 1999).

Kamphaus et al. (2006) identified the inability to adequately account for comorbidity as another main weakness of categorical classification systems. Studies have found that a large number of individuals meeting diagnostic criteria for one disorder also have at least one additional disorder (Clark et al. 1995; Wittchen 1996). This finding suggests that either psychopathology lends itself to high rates of co-occurring disorders or that the current diagnostic system does not adequately discriminate between disorders (Kamphaus et al. 2006). In either case, the current psychiatric systems of classification are not adequately addressing the issue of comorbidity.

The dimensional model does appear to solve many of the problems associated with categorical classification. Dimensional models provide clinicians with clinical symptom presentations of varying severity as well as those that may be considered subsyndromal or subthreshold, comorbid, or atypical in categorical classification systems. Kamphaus et al. (2006) identified a number of advantages of the dimensional model in comparison to the categorical model including better predictive validity and reliability (Cantwell 1996; Fergusson and Horwood 1995), a minimal need for clinical judgment and inference (Haynes and OBrien 1988), greater sensitivity in detecting comorbid conditions (Caron and Rutter 1991), the ability to depict multiple symptom patterns in a single individual simultaneously, and the opportunity to identify subtypes or clusters of individuals in order to guide the development of more efficient subtype-specific intervention and prevention services (Achenbach 1995; Bergman and Mangusson 1997).

Limitations of the dimensional model also exist; these limitations generally concern the lack of consensus amongst professionals and lack of supporting research available at this time. Information provided from dimensional methods is less concise and less familiar to professionals and therefore has the potential to hinder communication. Additionally, the statistics and computations necessary for dimensional methods may be too cumbersome and complicated, therefore lacking clinical utility and feasibility (Kamphaus et al. 2006).

Some researchers have suggested that categorical methods may be optimal for certain syndromes while dimensional methods would be better for others (Arend et al. 1996). Certain childhood disorders with symptoms that are distributed along continua in the population and are related to the internalizing and externalizing dimensions of psychopathology may be measured most effectively by using dimensional models. These disorders might include inattention, hyperactivity, conduct problems and oppositional behaviors, anxiety and somatization, depression, learning disabilities, and mental retardation (Kamphaus et al. 2006). Other disorders, such as schizophrenia, eating disorders, and autism appear to differ qualitatively from normality and are best identified using a more categorical approach.

Current Classification Systems

Diagnostic and Statistical Manual of Mental Disorders

The *Diagnostic and Statistical Manual of Mental Disorders*—Fifth Edition (DSM-V; APA 2013) is currently the most widely used method of psychiatric classification in the USA. Although largely categorical in nature, the latest version of the DSM has begun to incorporate aspects of the dimensional model into some of its disorders (i.e., mental retardation, attention deficit/hyperactivity disorder).

The first two editions of the DSM (1952, 1968) were developed using a categorical model of classification. The definitions of disorders centered around an underlying pathological core largely based upon Freud's psychodynamic theories. The

DSM-III (1980/1987), however, took a more "functional approach to viewing disorders in which mental disorders were viewed as a clinically significant behavioral or psychological syndrome or pattern that occurs in an individual and that is typically associated with either a painful symptom (distress) or impairment in one or more areas of functioning (disability)" (Kamphaus and Frick 2002, p. 53). Additionally, an emphasis was made to make diagnostic categories more empirical by basing classification on scientific evidence rather than clinical consensus (Blashfield 1998). Disorders were also defined more specifically, which led to greater reliability in the DSM-III and DSM-IV. Following the publication of the DSM-III, numerous studies began to appear in the literature exploring the validity of the diagnostic criteria, allowing for the development of a more comprehensive research base on which to develop the DSM-IV. However, reliability and validity of DSM diagnoses continues to be lower than that of most psychological tests (Sroufe 1997; Kamphaus et al. 2006).

The DSM-IV, published in 1994, contained 354 diagnostic categories nested within 17 major categories. It retained the multiaxial system from the DSM-III along which individuals should be coded:

- Axis I: Clinical disorders, other conditions that may be a focus of clinical attention (includes 16 general categories of disorders)
- Axis II: Personality disorders/mental retardation (includes 11 different personality disorders, and mental retardation)
- Axis III: General medical conditions (includes current general medical conditions that may be relevant in understanding or treating the individual's mental disorder)
- Axis IV: Psychosocial and environmental problems (includes psychosocial and environmental factors that may affect diagnosis, treatment, and prognosis of mental disorders)
- Axis V: Global assessment of functioning (includes a rating of overall level of functioning with 1 being most severe and 100 as most adaptive)

The newest edition of the DSM, the DSM-V, acknowledges the movement toward dimensional approaches to diagnosis. The dimensionality of broader internalizing and externalizing features are discussed in the introduction; furthermore, high levels of comorbidity are provided as evidence of the need to consider more dimensional approaches to diagnosis. The DSM-V (APA 2013) does not assume an underlying pathology and many of the diagnostic criteria of the disorders are based upon patterns of symptom covariation (e.g., ADHD)—a basic tenet of the dimensional model. Furthermore, the multiaxial approach to diagnosis has been dropped in this most recent edition, citing limited additional information in support of Axes III and IV and poor psychometric properties of the Global Assessment of Functioning score provided on Axis V. Despite consideration of a more dimensional method, the DSM-V remains consistent with the categorical approach, continuing to classify disorders into discrete categories and calls for additional information prior to changing most diagnoses.

Individuals with Disabilities Education Improvement Act (IDEIA)

In 1974, Public Law 94–142, or the Education of Handicapped Children's Act was implemented. The law required that the US public schools identify and serve all children with disabilities in the least restrictive environment possible, including those who had previously been educated in various alternative settings such as residential treatment programs. In 1986, an amendment was made to the act that added an early intervention program for children ages 0–2 and the inclusion of children ages 3–5 as eligible for free and appropriate public education. In 1990, another amendment changed the Education for All Handicapped Children Act to the Individuals with Disabilities Act (IDEA). The new amendment expanded special education categories to include autism and traumatic brain disorder and added transition services for children ages 16 and older.

Two reauthorizations of the act have since occurred, one in 1997 and most recently in 2004 when the name was changed to the IDEIA. Several issues were emphasized in the 2004 reauthorization including the reduction of overidentification of ethnically diverse populations, early intervention, streamlining of the special education process, as well as the introduction of alternative models, such as response to intervention (RtI), for classifying specific learning disabilities (see Chap. 5).

Although the IDEIA is legislation and not a formal diagnostic system, the implementation of its regulations has, in effect, created a diagnostic system that functions to classify individuals as eligible for special education or related services in the schools (Kamphaus et al. 2006). The DSM and IDEIA offer two very different perspectives on children's adjustment problems. The DSM-V focuses on identifying problematic patterns of behavior that cause suffering or obvious impairment in life adaptation. It is very broad by intention as the goal is to classify all significant problems of behavior and adjustment. IDEIA, on the other hand, focuses on identifying psychological or medical disabilities that would prevent a child or adolescent from benefiting fairly from a public education unless appropriate remediation is made. In general, the goal of DSM-V is aimed at reliable and valid classification for the purposes of clinical treatment and research to improve clinical treatment. IDEIA is aimed at providing safeguards so that all children and adolescents in the USA have a fair and equal opportunity to benefit from public education, and to ensure free and appropriate public education and related services to *all* children and adolescents with disabilities.

As part of this legislation, specific classification criteria for 12 disability conditions (see Table 2.2) eligible for special education were developed and adopted. This system can be considered another categorical classification system as students either meet criteria or do not.

The two categories most pertinent to this text and to emotional and behavior assessment are other health impairment (OHI) and emotional disturbance. Under IDEIA, ADHD is a medical condition, diagnosed by a medical doctor. Children with ADHD are served under the OHI special education category. To be classi-

Table 2.2 Disability classifications under IDEIA

Classifications under IDEIA
Autism
Specific learning disability
Intellectual disability
Emotional disturbance
Other health impairment
Speech–language impairment
Significant developmental delay
Deaf/blind
Deaf/hard of hearing
Visual impairment
Orthopedic impairment
Traumatic brain injury

fied as OHI, individuals must have "limited strength, vitality, or alertness including heightened alertness to environmental stimuli, that results in limited alertness with respect to the educational environment that:

1. Is due to chronic or acute health problems such as asthma, ADHD, diabetes, epilepsy, heart condition, hemophilia, lead poisoning, leukemia, nephritis, rheumatic fever, and sickle cell anemia
2. Adversely affects a student's educational performance."

The diagnostic criteria for emotional disturbance (see Table 2.3), developed by Eli Bower in 1968, have been controversial since their inception as they do not align with the DSM and are quite ambiguous, leaving considerable room for interpretation (Kamphaus et al. 2006).

Table 2.3 Criteria for emotional disturbance

Criteria for emotional disturbance under the Individuals with Disabilities Education Act (2004)
1. The term means a condition exhibiting one or more of the following characteristics over a long period of time and to a marked degree that adversely affects a child's educational performance:
A. An inability to learn that cannot be explained by intellectual, sensory, or health factors
B. An inability to build or maintain satisfactory interpersonal relationships with peers and teachers
C. Inappropriate types of behavior or feelings under normal circumstances
D. A general pervasive mood of unhappiness or depression
E. A tendency to develop physical symptoms or fears associated with personal or school problems
2. The term includes schizophrenia. The term does not apply to children who are socially maladjusted, unless determined that they have an emotional disturbance

Current Mental Health System Trends and Issues

The present state of child and adolescent mental health in the USA has become an area of major concern across the highest levels of government, including the president of the USA and members of both the House of Representatives and the Senate. In the past 15 years, a number of conferences and commissions have been formed in order to work toward the development of action plans and solutions to the problem at hand.

In 1999, the Substance Abuse and Mental Health Services Administration (SAMHSA) and the National Institutes of Health (NIH) collaborated in creating the *Report of the Surgeon General on Mental Health*. This report calls for the implementation of a public/community health model. According to the public health model, we should be focusing on strategies that affect the population at large, thus emphasizing health promotion, disease prevention, early detection, and universal access to care. In line with this model, the report identifies the following courses of action: continue to build the research base, overcome stigma, improve public awareness of effective treatments for mental health problems, ensure the supply of mental health services and providers, ensure delivery of state-of-the-art treatment, tailor treatment to age, gender, race, and culture where appropriate, facilitate entry into treatment, and reduce financial barriers to treatment (United States Department of Health and Human Services 1999). Of essential importance is that first-line contacts in the community, such as schools and primary care physicians, recognize and respond sensitively to mental illness, know what resources exist, and make proper referrals or address problems effectively themselves (United States Department of Health and Human Services 1999).

In 2000, the Department of Health and Human Services, Department of Education, and Department of Justice collaborated on a report about the Surgeon General's Conference on Children's Mental Health. In creating this report, they outlined eight goals for their national action agenda:

1. Promote public awareness of children's mental health issues and reduce stigma associated with mental illness.
2. Continue to develop, disseminate, and implement scientifically proven prevention and treatment services in the field of children's mental health.
3. Improve the assessment of and recognition of mental health needs in children.
4. Eliminate racial/ethnic and socioeconomic disparities in access to mental health-care services.
5. Improve the infrastructure for children's mental health services, including support for scientifically proven interventions across professions.
6. Increase access to and coordination of quality mental health-care services.
7. Train frontline providers to recognize and manage mental health issues, and educate mental health-care providers about scientifically-proven prevention and treatment services.
8. Monitor the access to and coordination of quality mental health-care services.

The steps that must be taken in order to reach these goals are numerous; however, many of these steps are in agreement with the public health model advocated by the SAMHSA and NIH in the preceding report. These steps include identifying early indicators for mental health problems, encouraging early identification of mental health needs in existing preschool, education, health, welfare, and substance abuse treatment systems, creating tangible tools for practitioners in these systems to help them assess children's social and emotional needs, training all primary health-care providers and educational personnel to recognize early indicators of mental health problems, and encouraging the health-care system to respond to mental health prevention and treatment service needs through universal and comprehensive health coverage (United States Public Health Service 2000).

In 2003, George W. Bush created the New Freedom Commission on Mental Health. Once again, goals were put forth for the transformed mental health system:

1. Americans understand that mental health is essential to overall health.
2. Mental health care is consumer and family driven.
3. Disparities in mental health services are eliminated.
4. Early mental health screening, assessment, and referral to services are common practice.
5. Excellent mental health care is delivered and research is accelerated.
6. Technology is used to access mental health care and information.

A common thread found in all of these action plans is the need for early identification of children and adolescents for mental health problems. For example, the *Report of the Surgeon General's Conference on Children's Mental Health* calls for screening and early identification of children within key service systems as well as the development of "a universal measurement system across all major service sectors that is age-appropriate, culturally competent, and gender sensitive to (i) identify children, including those with special health-care needs, who may need mental health services; (ii) track child progress during treatment; and (iii) measure treatment outcomes for individual patients" (United States Public Health Service 2000). Bush's 2003 New Freedom Commission on Mental Health (New Freedom Commission on Mental Health 2003) also advocates for early mental health screening, assessment, and referral to services, resulting in shorter and less disabling courses of impairment. It states that, "Quality screening and early intervention will occur in both readily accessible, low-stigma settings such as primary health-care facilities and schools, and in settings in which a high level of risk exists for mental health problems, such as criminal and juvenile justice and child welfare systems." Additionally, in 2002, the President's Commission on Excellence in Special Education put forth that:

> …compelling research sponsored by [the office of Special Education Programs] on emotional and behavioral difficulties indicates that children at risk for these difficulties could also be identified through universal screening and more significant disabilities prevented through classroom-based approaches involving positive discipline and classroom management. (Section 2, p. 2)

These action plans suggest that through universal screening for mental health concerns we can work to reduce risk, prevent onset, and intervene early so as to improve outcomes significantly.

In May 2005, the Campaign for Mental Health Reform addressed the US Senate and House of Representatives and referred to the current state of child and adolescent mental health services as a "public health crisis." To be convinced of the idea that we are in the midst of such a public health crisis, one must understand the importance of mental health to our overall well-being as well as the inadequacy of our current mental health system of care and prevention. In the next chapter, we discuss the current status of the mental health system and build the case for the importance of universal screening efforts to support early intervention and prevention efforts.

References

Achenbach, T. M. (1995). Developmental issues in assessment, taxonomy, and diagnosis of child and adolescent psychopathology. In D. Cicchetti & D. Cohen (Eds.), *Developmental psychopathology: Risk, disorder, and adaptation* (Vol. 2, pp. 715–752). New York: Wiley.

Achenbach, T. M., & McConaughy, S. H. (1992). Taxonomy of internalizing disorders of childhood and adolescence. In W. M. Reynolds (Ed.), *Internalizing disorders in children and adolescents* (pp. 19–60). New York: Wiley.

American Psychiatric Association. (1994). *Diagnostic and statistical manual of mental disorders* (4th Ed.), Washington, DC: American Psychiatric Association.

American Psychiatric Association. (2013). *Diagnostic and statistical manual of mental disorders* (5th Ed.). Washington, DC. American Psychiatric Association.

Aos, S., Lieb, R., Mayfield, J., Miller, M., & Pennucci, A. (2004). *Benefits and costs of prevention and early intervention programs for youth.* Olympia: Washington State Institute for Public Policy.

Arend, R., Lavigne, J. V., Rosenbaum, D., Binns, J. J., & Christoffel, K. K. (1996). Relation between taxonomicand quantitative diagnostic systems in preschool children: Emphasis on disruptive disorders. *Journal of Clinical Child Psychology, 25*(4), 388–397.

Baily, M. A., & Murray, T. H. (2008). Ethics, evidence, and cost in newborn screening. *Hastings Center Report, 38*, 23–31.

Bergman, L. R., & Magnusson, D. (1997). A person-oriented approach in research on developmental psychopathology. *Development and Psychopathology, 9*(2), 291–319.

Blashfield, R. K. (1998). Diagnostic models and systems. In A. S. Bellack, M. Hersen, & C. R. Reynolds (Eds.), *Comprehensive clinical psychology: Vol. 4. Assessment.* New York: Elsevier Science.

Brestan, E. V., & Eyberg, S. M. (1998) Effective psychosocial treatments of conduct-disordered children and adolescents: 29 years, 82 studies, and 5272 kids. *Journal of Clinical Child Psychology, 27*, 180–189.

Campaign for Mental Health Reform. (2005). A public health crisis: Children and adolescents with mental disorders. Congressional briefing. www.mhreform.org/kids. Accessed 1 Sept 2005.

Cantwell, D. P. (1996). Classification of child and adolescent psychopathology. *Journal of Child Psychology and Psychiatry, 37*, 3–12.

Caron, C., & Rutter, M. (1991). Comorbidity in child psychopathology: Concepts, issues, and research strategies. *Journal of Child Psychology and Psychiatry and Allied Disciplines, 32*, 1063–1080.

Catranis, T. (2005). New Pap smear guidelines. www.nbc15online.com. Accessed 24 July 2008.

Chandler, L. A. (1990). The projective hypothesis and the development of projective techniques for children. In C. R. Reynolds & R. W. Kamphaus (Eds.), *Handbook of psychological and educational assessment of children: Personality, behavior, & context* (pp. 55–69). New York: Guilford Press.

Clark, L. A., Watson, D., & Reynolds, W. S. (1995). Diagnosis and classification of psychopathology: Challenges to the current system and future directions. *Annual Review of Psychology, 46*, 121.

Dever, B. V., & Kamphaus, R. W. (2013). Social and emotional assessment of children in schools. In K. F. Geisinger, B. A. Bracken, J. F. Carlson, J. C. Hansen, N. R. Kuncel, S. P. Reise, & M. C. Rodriguez (Eds.). *APA Handbook of Testing and Assessment. Vol. 3: Testing and Assessment in School Psychology and Education* (pp. 129–148). Washington, DC: American Psychological Association.

Dowdy, E., Mays, K. L., Kamphaus, R. W., & Reynolds, C. R. (2009). Roles of diagnosis and classification in school psychology. In T. B. Gutkin & C. R. Reynolds (Eds.), *The handbook of school psychology* (4th ed., pp. 191–209). Hoboken: Wiley.

DuBois, P. H., & Garson, E. (1970). *A history of psychological testing*. Boston. Allyn and Bacon.

Edelbrock, C. (1979). Empirical classification of children's behavior disorders: Progress based on parent and teacher ratings. *School Psychology Digest, 8*, 355–369.

Fergusson, D.M., & Horwood, J. (1995). Predictive validity of categorically and dimensionally scored measures of disruptive childhood behaviors. *Journal of the American Academy of Child and Adolescent Psychiatry, 34*, 477–487.

Fletcher, J. M. (1985). External validation of learning disability typologies. In B. P. Rourke (Ed.), *Neuropsychology of learning disabilities: Essentials of subtype analysis* (pp. 187–211). New York: Guilford Press.

French, J. L., & Hale, R. L. (1990). A history of the development of psychological and educational testing. In C. R. Reynolds & R. W. Kamphaus (Eds.), *Handbook of psychological and educational assessment of children: Intelligence and achievement* (pp. 3–28). New York: Guilford Press.

Harting, D., & Glenn, B. (1951). A comparison of blood-sugar and urine-sugar determinations for the detection of diabetes. *The New England Journal of Medicine, 245*, 48–54.

Hathaway, S. R., & McKinney, J. C. (1942). *Minnesota multiphasic personality inventory*. Minneapolis: University of Minnesota Press.

Haynes, S. N., & O'Brien, W. H. (1988). The Gordian knot of DSM-III use: Integrating principles of behavior classification and complex causal models. *Behavioral Assessment, 10*, 95–105.

Hudziak, J. J., Wadsworth, M. E., Heath, A. C., & Achenbach, T. M. (1999). Latent class analysis of child behavior checklist attention problems. *Journal of the American Academy of Child and Adolescent Psychiatry, 38*, 985–991.

Individuals with Disabilities Education Act of 1990 (IDEA), P.L. 101–476. (1990).

Individuals with Disabilities Education Improvement Act, 20 U.S.C. § 1400. (2004).

Jablensky, A. (1999). The nature of psychiatric classification: Issues beyond ICD-10 and DSM-IV. *Australian and New Zealand Journal of Psychiatry, 33*, 137–144.

Johnson, P. C., & Farnie, M. A. (1994). Testing for syphilis. *Dermatologic clinics, 12*, 9–17.

Kamphaus, R. W., & Frick, P. J. (2002). *Clinical assessment of child and adolescent personality and behavior* (2nd ed.). Boston: Allyn & Bacon.

Kamphaus, R. W., Rowe, E. W., Dowdy, E. T., & Henry, C. N. (2006) Classification and diagnosis concepts. In R. W. Kamphaus & J. M. Campbell (Eds.), *Psychodiagnostic assessment of children: Dimensional and categorical approaches* (pp. 1–27). New Jersey: Wiley.

Kaslow, N. J., & Thompson, M. P. (1998). Applying the criteria for empirically supported treatments to studies of psychosocial interventions for child and adolescent depression. *Journal of Clinical Child Psychology, 27*, 146–155.

Kleinmuntz, B. (1967). *Personality measurement: An introduction*. Homewood: Dorsey Press.

Kraepelin, E. (1902/1896). *Clinical psychiatry: A text-book for students and physicians* (6th ed., translated by A. R. Diefendorf). London: Macmillan.

Larsen, S. A., Steiner, B. M., & Rudolph, A. H. (1995). Laboratory diagnosis and interpretation of tests for syphilis. *Clinical Microbiology Reviews, 8*(1), 1–21.

Law, P. (1975). Law 94–142. *Education for all Handicapped Children Act, 20*, 1401–1461.

Lee C. M., Huxley D. R., Lam T. H., et al. (2007). Prevalence of diabetes mellitus and population attributable fractions for coronary heart disease and stroke mortality in the WHO South-East Asia and Western Pacific regions. *Asia Pacific journal of clinical nutrition, 16*, 187–92.

Martin, R.P. (1988). *Assessment of personality and behavior problems: Infancy through adolescence*. New York: Guilford Press.

Morabia, A. & Zhang, F.F. (2004). History of medical screening: From concepts to action. *Postgraduate Medical Journal, 80*, 463–469.

Moyer, V. A., Calonge, N., Teutsch, S. M., & Botkin, J. R. (2008). Expanding newborn screening: Process, policy, and priorities. *Hastings Center Report, 38*, 32–39.

New Freedom Commission on Mental Health (2003). *Achieving the promise: Transforming mental health care in America, final report*. DHHS Pub. No. SMA-0303832. Rockville, MD. http://www.mentalhealthcommission.gov/. Accessed 1 Sept 2005.

Patten S. F. J. (1969). Diagnostic cytology of the uterine cervix. In G.L. Wied, E.V. Haam, & L.G. Koss (Eds.), *Manographs in clinical cytology*. Baltimore: Williams & Wilkins.

Pelham, W. E. Jr., Wheeler, T., & Chronis, A. (1998) Empirically supported psychosocial treatments for attention deficit hyperactivity disorder. *Journal of Clinical Child Psychology, 27*, 190–205.

Reynolds, C. R., & Kamphaus, R. W. (1992). *Behavior Assessment System for Children (BASC)*. Circle Pines: Pearson.

Reynolds, C. R., & Kamphaus, R. W. (2004). *Behavior Assessment System for Children-Second Edition (BASC-2)*. Circle Pines: Pearson.

Seal, K. H., Bertenthal, D., Maguen, S., Gima, K., Chu, A., & Marmar, C. R. (2008). Getting beyond "Don't Ask, Don't Tell": an evaluation of US veterans administration postdeployment mental health screening of veterans returning from Iraq and Afghanistan. *Research and Practice, 98*, 714–720.

Smith R. A., Saslow D., Sawyer K. A., Burke W., Costanza M. E., Evans W. P. III, Foster R. S. Jr, Hendrick E., Eyre H. J., Sener S. American Cancer Society High-Risk Work Group, American Cancer Society Screening Older Women Work Group, American Cancer Society Mammography Work Group, American Cancer Society Physical Examination Work Group, American Cancer Society New Technologies Work Group, & American Cancer Society Breast Cancer Advisory Group. (2003). American Cancer Society guidelines for breast cancer screening: update 2003. *CA: A Cancer Journal for Clinicians, 53*, 138–40.

Sroufe, L. A. (1997). Psychopathology as an outcome of development. *Developmental Psychopathology, 9*(2), 251–268.

Stone, M., Merikangas, K. R., Leckman, J. F., Zhang, H., & Kasl, S. (1999). Psychosocial and clinical correlates of ADHD in a community sample of school-age children. *Journal of the American Academy of Child and Adolescent Psychiatry, 38*, 976–984.

Tupes, E. C, & Christal, R. E. (1961). Recurrent personality factors based on trait ratings (USAF ASD Tech. Rep. No. 61–97). Lackland Air Force Base, TX: US Air Force.

United States Department of Health and Human Services (1999). *Mental Health: A Report of the Surgeon General*. Rockville, MD: US Department of Health and Human Services, Substance abuse, and Mental Health Services Administration, Center for Mental Health Services, National Institutes of Health, National Institute of Mental Health. http://www.surgeongeneral.gov/library/mentalhealth/home.html. Accessed 1 Sept 2005.

United States Public Health Service (2000). *Report of the Surgeon General's Conference on Children's Mental Health: A national action agenda*. Washington D.C.: Department of Health and Human Services. http://www.surgeongeneral.gov/topics/cmh/childreport.htm. Accessed 1 Sept 2005.

United States Preventive Services Task Force (2008). Diabetes Mellitus (Type 2) in Adults: Screening. http://www.uspreventiveservicestaskforce.org/Page/Topic/recommendation-summary/diabetes-mellitus-type-2-in-adults-screening. Accessed 26 June 2015.

Watson, M. S., Mann, M. Y., Lloyd-Puryear, M. A., Rinaldo, P., & Howell, R. R. (2006). Newborn screening: Towards a uniform screening panel and system. *Genetics in Medicine, 8*, S12–S252.

Wilson J. M. & Jungner, F. (1968). *Principles and practices of screening for diseases*. Geneva: WHO.

Wittchen, H. U. (1996). What is comorbidity: Fact or artifact? *British Journal of Psychiatry, 168*, 7–8.

Woodworth, R. S. (1918). *Personal data sheet*. Chicago: Stoelting.

Chapter 3
Current Systems of Identification and the Case for Mental Health Screening

Importance of Mental Health in Children

Evidence abounds that emotional and behavioral adjustment in children is intertwined with their general physical health and academic achievement, and has also been linked to successful adaptation throughout their lives (Masten and Coatsworth 1998). Mental disorders rank first among illnesses that cause disability in the USA, Canada, and Western Europe (New Freedom Commission on Mental Health 2003). In the USA, mental illness accounts for more than 15 % of the overall burden of disease (United States Department of Health and Human Services 1999). Suicide has also been found to be a major problem worldwide, emerging as the third leading cause of death in youth aged 15–24. Over 90 % of children and adolescents who commit suicide have at least one mental disorder (Campaign for Mental Health Reform 2005).

As anyone who works in a school can tell you, the behaviors and needs of children at risk for or with emotional and behavioral problems are highly demanding and can easily overwhelm the resources of the schools. It is estimated that students with the most severe emotional and behavioral disorders constitute between 1 and 5 % of the school population but consume more that 50 % of time and resources of teachers and administrators (U.S. Public Health Service 2000).

Research has also demonstrated that the effects of emotional and behavioral disorders in children, as well as the disorders themselves, tend to persist into adulthood with 74 % of 21-year-olds with mental disorders having had prior mental health problems (Aronen et al. 1999; United States Public Health Service 2000). Children with emotional and behavioral problems are more likely to drop out of school, abuse substances, be involved in the juvenile justice system, and commit suicide. Strikingly, approximately 50 % of students aged 14 and older with a mental disorder will drop out of school; only 42 % of those who remain in school will graduate with a diploma (United States Public Health Service 2000). Additionally, 65 % of boys and 75 % of girls in juvenile detention centers have at least one mental disorder (Campaign for Mental Health Reform 2005).

M. C. Stiffler, B. V. Dever, *Mental Health Screening at School*, Contemporary Issues in Psychological Assessment, DOI 10.1007/978-3-319-19171-3_3

The cost to society is high not only in human terms, but in financial terms as well. Mental disorders account for between 5% and 10% of the total cost and morbidity burden due to disease (Jenkins 1998). In the USA, the indirect cost of mental illness is about $79 billion annually. This figure includes costs due to loss of productivity, incarceration, and treatment. When children with untreated emotional and behavioral disorders become adults, they continue to utilize more health-care services and incur much higher health-care costs than other adults. The states spend nearly $1 billion per year on medical costs associated with completed suicides and suicide attempts by youth (Campaign for Mental Health Reform 2005). Cohen (1998) found that diverting just one at-risk child from developing serious conduct problems may result in a savings of nearly $2 million to society.

Early emotional and behavioral difficulties, including subsyndromal symptomatology, can lead to a pattern of adjustment problems that may be transient or long standing, depending on the services provided and the timing of these services. The longer a child's emotional and behavioral problems go unidentified, the more stable his or her maladaptive trajectory is likely to be. As such, early identification and intervention for youth with emotional and behavioral problems can help to minimize the long-term detriment and reduce the overall health-care burden and costs of mental disorders. Hester et al. (2004; p. 5) concluded that early identification and intervention for students at risk for emotional and behavior disorders appears to be the "most powerful course of action for ameliorating life-long problems associated with children at risk."

When children are young, they exhibit more plasticity and malleability both behaviorally and neurodevelopmentally, thus making them more responsive and their maladaptive behaviors easier to modify (Hirshfield-Becker and Biederman 2002; Bailey et al. 1999). Early identification and intervention also catches developing problems before they become more severe or expand into numerous co-occurring disorders. Untreated emotional and behavioral problems during this crucial time tend to persist into later childhood and adulthood. These problems interfere with the development of critical emotional and cognitive skills, escalate in severity, and lead to a downward spiral of school failure, unemployment, substance abuse, and poverty (Hirshfield-Becker and Biederman 2002; McGoey et al. 2002; United States Public Health Service 2000). Walker et al. (1995) suggested that if antisocial behavior is not corrected by the third grade, it will persist and must be managed as a chronic condition. Through early identification and treatment, we may prevent negative lifelong outcomes. Therefore, childhood is an essential time to identify and prevent chronic mental disorders as well as promote healthy development. In order to so, children must be accurately identified as at-risk and provided services early.

Current Mental Health-Care System

The current mental health-care system has little chance of succeeding; it fails at the outset by not identifying children in need of services. Recent research indicates that approximately 20% of children have a diagnosable mental disorder; furthermore,

10–13 % of preschoolers, aged 1–6, have emotional or behavioral disorders (Campaign for Mental Health Reform 2005; Friedman et al. 1996). Thus, many of these problems begin early in life and are ignored. For example, Fantuzzo et al. (2003) found that the Head Start staff under-identified children with behavioral or emotional problems and children with the highest risk of poor academic readiness were likely to be unidentified and untreated.

In general, only 15–20 % of children with emotional and behavioral problems receive any type of mental health services in a given year (Ringel and Sturm 2001; United States Public Health Service 2000). Jenkins (1998) estimated that mental health specialists are able to meet the needs of only 10 % of all children with emotional and behavioral problems. Generally, the children who do receive services are those with the most fully developed and severe mental disorders. However, children who exhibit signs of risk or subsyndromal symptomatology also need access to interventions in order to prevent the development of more serious disorders. Thus, although the most effective way to maximize the likelihood of positive treatment outcomes is to identify and treat children early, children must often wait until their problems are "serious enough" before they can receive services; this is often referred to as the "Wait-to-Fail" approach.

The median lag between the onset of a mental disorder and the start of treatment is about 10 years. Disorders emerging in childhood have the longest delays in treatment, perhaps due to reliance on parents or other adults as informants (National Mental Health Association, 2005). A critical gap exists between those who need mental health services and those who actually receive them. This unmet need for services remains as high today as it was 20 years ago (United States Public Health Service 2000).

A recent review of the literature by Jamieson and Romer (2005) called for a national effort to reorganize current mental health identification processes through the following observation:

> Because it is clear that early detection and referral for treatment should be a high national priority, it is disappointing to learn from research conducted as part of the commissions (referring to expert panels created as part of the Adolescent Mental Health Initiative of the Annenberg Foundation Trust) that the primary care system and schools are inadequately prepared to meet this challenge. As a result, schools do not intervene until illnesses progress and come to the attention of staff (p. 619).

Potential Settings for Mental Health Identification

Primary care and school settings appear to be two of the most important systems for the potential early detection of emotional and behavioral problems in children and adolescents. The majority of children are seen in these settings, thus providing the opportunity to reach large numbers of youth. A number of challenges exist, however, that contribute to the failure of these settings to identify and treat children with emotional and behavioral problems.

Health-Care Settings

In primary care settings, we first must address the problem of access to medical care. Despite the recent strides that have been made, many adults and children in the US population do not have health insurance. Additionally, disparity exists in insurance coverage of general health versus mental health services. In fact, studies show that the gap in insurance coverage between mental health and other health services is widening (United States Department of Health and Human Services 1999). Therefore, even those who have private health insurance may find it difficult to finance mental health services.

Second, the stigma of mental disorders still exists in our society and deters Americans from seeking care. In order to move past the stigma of seeking treatment for mental health disorders, it is critical to engage in conversations about these issues early and often with the entire population, rather than seeking only to assign labels and diagnoses to a select few.

Furthermore, parents are often unaware that they can discuss mental health issues with primary care physicians; parents tend to assume that primary care physicians are only concerned with physical health. There is also some evidence to suggest that parents are more likely to seek services for their children when they exhibit behaviors such as hyperactivity and aggression rather than internalizing symptomatology such as anxiety (Arcia and Fernandez 2003).

Lastly, there tends to be poor recognition of mental illness by physicians due to time limitations, limited training in mental health issues, and a focus on the central task of assessing physical health. The average visit with a primary care physician is only between 11 and 15 minutes (United States Department of Health and Human Services 1999). Although primary care providers are identifying an increasing number of emotional and behavioral problems (15–30 %), rates of recognition (48–57 %) are still low and referrals to mental health specialists are unlikely (United States Department of Health and Human Services 1999).

The pediatric emergency department is another medical setting where there is potential to identify children with mental health issues. On average, children seen in the emergency department are more likely to be exposed to risk factors such as poverty, abuse, and family mental health problems. In addition, suicidal children and adolescents often seek medical care prior to suicide attempts, making the emergency department an important venue for mental health screening (Williams et al. 2011). Although time is most frequently cited as a critical barrier to mental health screening in this setting, the vast majority of parents (82 %), children (75 %), doctors (99 %), and nurses (97 %) found screening to be acceptable and feasible when conducted during emergency room visits (Williams et al. 2011). This suggests that the pediatric emergency department is a promising venue for early identification of mental health problems.

School-Based Settings

Perhaps due to the captive audience of children and adolescents, the school is the most common place for mental health service delivery (O'Connell et al. 2009; U.S. Department of Health and Human Services 1999). Unfortunately, the current model of referral for mental health services in schools has failed to result in improvements in the rates of mental illness. As stated previously, approximately 20 % of school-age children and adolescents are experiencing symptomology that would qualify them for a psychiatric diagnosis, and this estimate remains largely unchanged over time (Costello et al. 2003); however, the majority of these students are never identified for service delivery (Dowdy et al. 2010; Mills et al. 2006). A part of the challenge is the current "Wait-to-Fail" approach of service delivery that often does not utilize the skill set of school psychologists and other mental health professionals in schools until a student has reached the threshold of qualification for services or diagnosis.

In schools, children with emotional and behavioral needs are usually identified only after their regular classroom teachers cannot manage their problems. Most identification is done through teacher-initiated referral for evaluation—an idiosyncratic method that allows many children with emotional and behavioral, especially internalizing, problems to fall through the cracks (Eklund et al. 2009). Lloyd et al. (1991) found that 79 % of all school referrals involve general education teachers. Several studies have indicated that those students who are referred usually exhibit externalizing behavior problems that are highly disruptive and aversive to both teachers and peers (Grosenick 1981; Noel 1982) rather than internalizing problems such as depression, shyness, phobias, or social avoidance (Walker, Severson, Stiller, Williams, Haring, Shinn, & Todis 1988). Even if a child is referred, a series of parent conferences, discipline referrals, and trial interventions in the regular classroom often precede an actual referral for mental health services. As teacher training and understanding regarding issues of mental health varies widely, teacher referral may not be the most efficient method of identifying students who would benefit from intervention (Tilly, 2008).

Although most teachers likely have the best interests of their students in mind when making a decision to refer for mental health services, teacher referrals tend to conflict with data-driven approaches to identifying students' potential behavioral and emotional needs using standardized assessment instruments (Raines et al. 2012; Eklund et al. 2009); teacher reports tend to identify externalizing behaviors better than internalizing or emotional needs. Additionally, teacher referrals for services have been linked to the disproportionality of particular groups being referred for and receiving services. Disproportionality is defined as an overrepresentation or underrepresentation of a particular student group within a setting or outcome of interest, given that group's proportion in the total population. This overrepresentation is problematic if the services provided are not meeting the needs of, or are actually harming, those students (Algozzine 2005; Hosp and Reschly 2003). Unfortunately, this appears to be the case with the current mental health-care system in schools as the academic outcomes associated with the receipt of education services for emotional or behavioral problems are fairly dismal, including lower levels of achievement across academic subjects and higher rates of dropouts (e.g., Bradley et al. 2008; Greenbaum et al. 1996; Wagner et al. 2005).

Overall, African American students and males are the most likely to be overrepresented as a result of teacher referral for mental health services. African American students are overrepresented in special education, particularly in the categories of intellectual disability (ID) and emotional disturbance (ED; Ahram et al. 2011; Hosp and Reschly 2003; Jasper and Bouck 2013; MacMillan and Reschly 1998; Skiba et al. 2005, 2006b, 2008). In most studies, African American students are also more likely than their peers to be placed in more restrictive environments (Serwatka et al. 1995; Skiba et al. 2008); this disproportionality is most apparent among students with mild disabilities (Skiba et al. 2006a).

Similarly, males receiving special education services spend more time outside of general education settings than females receiving special education services, who are more often integrated into the general education classroom (Hosp and Reschly 2002), and are particularly at risk of being over-referred for behavioral problems (Bryan et al. 2012; Coutinho and Oswald 2005; Wallace et al. 2008). Unfortunately, the under-referral of females may be as problematic as the over-referral of males; research has indicated that females are typically older and suffer from greater levels of disability by the time they are identified for services (Gottlieb 1987; Wehmeyer and Schwartz 2001) as females do not present with behavioral problems that are disruptive to the classroom as frequently as males.

Improving Service Delivery

The current mental health service delivery system could be improved by adopting a more unified system of health care where children are served at a central location rather than the fragmented system that exists today in which children are vastly under-identified for services. Many researchers and clinicians (Huang et al. 2005; Tolan and Dodge 2005) have begun to advocate for a "systems of care" approach to mental health service delivery for children that embraces principles such as "wrapping services around the child rather than requiring the child to conform to the provider's culture and construal of care" and "including all service providers in a unified plan" (Tolan and Dodge 2005, p. 608). This approach essentially states that mental health services should be provided in settings where children are already seen, such as primary care and educational settings, thereby increasing the accessibility of these services for parents and children.

Schools appear to be optimal settings in which to access, assess, and intervene in the mental health of children. In primary care and emergency settings there is no guarantee that a particular child will be seen, especially when they are at risk or just beginning to exhibit symptoms. However, all school-age children in the USA are served by an education system. Schools are also an ideal location at which to observe children in their natural setting and have access to multiple informants (parents, multiple teachers, principals, and the students themselves). Schools are "where the children are" and therefore provide an optimal setting for service delivery.

More schools are beginning to provide school-based health centers that offer a one-stop source for medical, psychological, and preventative care. According to the National Assembly on School-Based Health Care (NASBHC), the number of such centers has increased from 120 sites in 1988 to more than 1500 in 2005 (Martin 2005). This involvement of the education system in the mental health of children is consistent with the current legislative demands such as No Child Left Behind (2002) in that the emotional and behavioral problems in children have been found to have a significant adverse effect on academic achievement (Gutman et al. 2003; Huang et al. 2005; Jimerson et al. 1999; McEvoy and Welker 2000; Rapport et al. 2001).

Universal Screening of Emotional and Behavioral Adjustment

A data-driven, empirical approach to referral that includes a universal screening program as the first step might assist efforts to both correctly identify students who are in need of mental health services in the schools earlier and decrease the overrepresentation of African American and male students in intervention programs. Universal emotional and behavioral screening is a quick and efficient way to assess a large number of children, identify children at risk of specific illnesses and disorders, and intervene early so as to significantly improve outcomes by reducing risk and preventing the onset of diagnosable disorders. This is especially true in the school context where there is universal access to children as a population. Jones, Dodge, Foster, Nix, and the Conduct Problems Prevention Research Group (2002) found that an inexpensive screening tool implemented in kindergarten accurately predicted which children would be receiving mental health, special education, or juvenile justice services 6 years later. Additionally, VanDerHeyden et al. (2003) demonstrated that universal screening using curriculum-based measurement probes and brief interventions resulted in fewer false positive identifications of students referred for special education when compared to teacher referral.

Tilly (2008, p. 31) drew the "conclusion that universal screening must become a part of business as usual in our schools." Unfortunately, emotional and behavioral screening for children and adolescents is currently minimal to nonexistent throughout the USA. Only 2–13 % of schools screen for emotional and behavioral problems (Bruhn et al. 2014; Romer and McIntosh 2005) and routine developmental and psychosocial assessments of young children in pediatric settings using standardized instruments are just as rare (United States Public Health Service 2000). As Huang stated, "By avoiding this, we are perpetuating stigma and failing to normalize mental health and recognize it as a critical part of overall health and well-being" (Campaign for Mental Health Reform 2005).

One reason that universal screening has not been properly integrated into service delivery in general, and in school settings in particular, is that there exists a lack of information that permits universal screening to be carried out feasibly and with fidelity. Dever et al. (2012) review common barriers to the implementation of universal screening, including time, cost, and difficulties making decisions among the multiple screening methods that are available. With all the responsibilities of school personnel, it is understandable that screening every child in a school or district might appear to be a daunting task.

However, school- and district-wide universal mental health screening is not only feasible, it is a necessary first step to a data-based decision-making process for identification and intervention purposes (Dever et al. 2013; Dever et al. 2012). Not only are the results of universal screening useful for individual-level decision-making and intervention planning, these data can be aggregated to the school- or district-level to provide more information about larger systems changes or prevention efforts that might be the most useful (Dever et al. 2013). Just as the surveillance of specific mental health disorders are critical to population-based public health efforts (Perou et al. 2013), the surveillance of overall risk of behavioral and emotional difficulties that is gathered during a universal screening program is critical to mental health efforts in schools (Dowdy et al. 2010).

The remainder of this book is structured to assist practitioners and researchers in making decisions about mental health screening, particularly in the school setting. First, those interested in screening must decide for what they will screen; more specifically, the decision must be made on whether to screen for overall mental health or risk of difficulties versus screening for specific disorders. This decision is one to be made based on the needs and goals of the particular school or district in question. Chapter 4 provides an overview of both broad and specific screening instruments that are currently available, including psychometric evidence. Second, if multiple forms are available, those interested in screening must determine who might be the best informant given the goals and limitations of the screening program; Chapter 6 presents information that we hope will assist with that decision. For those familiar with the Response to Intervention (RtI) approach to mental health service delivery, Chapter 5 explains how screening fits within this framework. Chapter 7 presents a case example of the implementation of universal screening in a school district for those readers who are interested in reflections from a real-world universal screening program. Finally, Chapter 8 outlines current issues and future directions for mental health screening, which are critical for both the practitioner and the researcher to consider when embarking upon work in the field.

References

Ahram, R., Fergus, E., & Noguera, P. (2011). Addressing racial/ethnic disproportionality in special education: Case studies of suburban school districts. *Teachers College Record, 113*(10), 2233–2266.

Algozzine, B. (2005). Restrictiveness and race in special education: Facts that remain difficult to ignore anymore. *Learning Disabilities: A Contemporary Journal, 3*(1), 64–69.

Arcia, E. & Fernandez, M. C. (2003). Presenting problems and assigned diagnoses among young Latino children with disruptive behavior. *Journal of Attention Disorders, 6,* 177–185.
Aronen, E. T., Teerikangas, O. M., & Kurkela, S. A. (1999). The continuity of psychiatric symptoms from adolescence into young adulthood. *Nordic Journal of Psychiatry, 53*(5), 333–338.
Bailey, D. B., Aytch, L. S., Odom, S. L., Symons, F., & Wolery, M. (1999). Early intervention as we know it. *Journal of Early Intervention, 24,* 1–14.
Bradley, R., Doolittle, J., & Bartolotta, R. (2008). Building on the data and adding to the discussion: The experiences and outcomes of students with emotional disturbance. *Journal of Behavioral Education, 17*(1), 4–23.
Bruhn, A. L., Woods-Groves, S., & Huddle, S. (2014). A preliminary investigation of emotional and behavioral screening practices in K-12 schools. *Education and Treatment of Children, 37,* 611–634.
Bryan, J., Day-Vines, N. L., Griffin, D., & Moore-Thomas, C. (2012). The disproportionality dilemma: Patterns of teacher referrals to school counselors for disruptive behavior. *Journal of Counseling & Development, 90*(2), 177–190.
Campaign for Mental Health Reform. (2005). A public health crisis: Children and adolescents with mental disorders. Congressional briefing. Retrieved September 1, 2005, from www.mhreform.org/kids.
Cohen, M. A. (1998). The monetary value of saving a high risk youth. *Journal of Quantitative Criminology, 4,* 5–33.
Costello, E. J., Mustillo, S., Erkanli, A., Keeler, G., & Angold, A. (2003). Prevalence and development of psychiatric disorders in childhood and adolescence. *Archives of General Psychiatry,* 60, 837–844.
Coutinho, M. J., & Oswald, D. P. (2005). State variation in gender disproportionality in special education findings and recommendations. *Remedial and Special Education, 26*(1), 7–15.
Dever, B. V., Kamphaus, R. W., Dowdy, E., Raines, T. C., & DiStefano, C. (2013). Surveillance of middle and high school mental health risk by student self-report screener. *Western Journal of Emergency Medicine, 14*(4), 384–390.
Dever, B. V., Raines, T. C., & Barclay, C. M. (2012). Chasing the unicorn: Practical implementation of universal screening for behavioral and emotional risk. *School Psychology Forum, 6*(4).
Dowdy, E., Ritchey, K., & Kamphaus, R. (2010). School-based screening: A population-based approach to inform and monitor children's mental health needs. *School Mental Health, 2*(4), 166–176.
Eklund, K., Renshaw, T. L., Dowdy, E., Jimerson, S. R., Hart, S. R., Jones, C. N., & Earhart, J. (2009). Early identification of behavioral and emotional problems in youth: Universal screening versus teacher-referral identification. *The California School Psychologist, 14*(1), 89–95.
Fantuzzo, J., Bulotsky, R., McDermott, P., Mosca, S., & Lutz, M. N. (2003). A multivariate analysis of emotional and behavioral adjustment and preschool educational outcomes. *School Psychology Review, 32,* 185–203.
Friedman, R. M., Katz-Leavy, J., Manderscheid, R., & Sondheimer, D. (1996). Prevalence of serious emotional disturbance in children and adolescents. In R. W. Manderscheid & M. A. Sonnenschein (Eds.), *Mental Health, United States, 1996* (pp. 71–88). Rockville: Center for Mental Health Services.
Gottlieb, B. W. (1987). *Gender differences in cognitive profiles among urban children placed in special education.* (ERIC Document Reproduction Service No. ED387972).
Greenbaum, P. E., Dedrick, R. F., Friedman, R. M., Kutash, K., Brown, E. C., Lardieri, S. P., & Pugh, A. M. (1996). National adolescent and child treatment study (NACTS): outcomes for children with serious emotional and behavioral disturbance. *Journal of Emotional and Behavioral Disorders, 4,* 130–146.
Grosenick, J. K. (1981). Public school and mental health services to severely behavior disordered students. *Behavior Disorders, 6,* 183–190.
Gutman, L. M., Sameroff, A. J., & Cole, R. (2003). Academic growth curve trajectories from 1st grade to 12th grade: Effects of multiple social risks and preschool child factors. *Developmental Psychology, 39,* 777–790.

Hester, P. P., Baltodano, H. M., Hendrickson, J. M., Tomelson, S. W., Conroy, M. A., & Gable, R. A. (2004). Lessons learned from research on early intervention: What teachers can do to prevent children's behavior problems. *Preventing School Failure, 49,* 5–10.

Hirshfield-Becker, D. R. & Biederman, J. (2002). Rationale and principles for early intervention with young children at risk for anxiety disorders. *Clinical Child and Family Psychology Review, 5,* 161–172.

Hosp, J. L., & Reschly, D. J. (2002). Regional differences in school psychology practice. *School Psychology Review, 31*(1), 11–29.

Hosp, J. L., & Reschly, D. J. (2003). Referral rates for intervention or assessment a meta-analysis of racial differences. *The Journal of Special Education, 37*(2), 67–80.

Huang, L., Stroul, B., Friedman, R., Mrazek, P., Friesen, B., Pires, S., & Mayberg, S. (2005). Transforming mental health care for children and their families. *American Psychologist, 60,* 615–627.

Jamieson, K. H. & Romer, D. (2005). A call to action on adolescent mental health. In D. L. Evans, E. B. Foa, R. E. Gur, H. Hendin, C. P. O'Brien, M. E. P. Seligman, & B. T. Walsh (Eds.), *Treating and preventing adolescent mental health disorders: What we know and what we don't know* (pp. 598–615). New York: Oxford University Press.

Jasper, A. D., & Bouck, E. C. (2013). Disproportionality among African American students at the secondary level: Examining the MID disability category. *Education and Training in Autism and Developmental Disabilities, 48*(1), 31–40.

Jenkins, R. (1998). Mental health and primary care—implications for policy. *International Review of Psychiatry, 10,* 158–160.

Jimerson, S., Egeland, A. B., & Teo, A. (1999). A longitudinal study of achievement trajectories: Factors associated with change. *Journal of Educational Psychology, 91,* 116–126.

Jones, D., Dodge, K. A., Foster, E. M., Nix, R., the Conduct Problems Prevention Research Group. (2002). Early identification of children at risk for costly mental health service use. *Prevention Science, 3,* 247–256.

Lloyd, J. W., Kauffman, J. M., Landrum, T. J., & Roe, D. L. (1991). Why do teachers refer pupils for special education: An analysis of referral records. *Exceptionality, 2,* 115–126.

MacMillan, D. L., & Reschly, D. J. (1998). Overrepresentation of minority students the case for greater specificity or reconsideration of the variables examined. *The Journal of Special Education, 32*(1), 15–24.

Martin, S. (2005). Healthy kids make better kids. *Monitor on Psychology, 36,* 24–26.

Masten, A. S. & Coatsworth, J. D. (1998). The development of competence in favorable and unfavorable environments: Lessons from research on successful children. *American Psychologist, 53,* 205–220.

McEvoy, A., & Welker, R. (2000). Antisocial behavior, academic failure, and school climate: A critical review. *Journal of Emotional and Behavioral Disorders, 8,* 130–141.

McGoey, K. E., Eckert, T. L., & Dupaul, G. J. (2002). Early intervention for preschool-age children with ADHD: A literature review. *Journal of Emotional and Behavioral Disorders, 10,* 1–27.

Mills, C., Stephan, S. H., Moore, E., Weist, M. D., Daly, B. P., & Edwards, M. (2006). The President's New Freedom Commission: Capitalizing on opportunities to advance school-based mental health services. *Clinical Child and Family Psychology Review, 9*(3), 149–161.

National Mental Health Association. (2005). Study shows mental illness often begins in youth, treatment delays worsen issues. *The Bell: The newsletter of the National Mental Health Association,* July 2005, 1–5.

New Freedom Commission on Mental Health. (2003). *Achieving the promise: Transforming mental health care in America, final report.* DHHS Pub. No. SMA—0303832. Rockville, MD. Retrieved September 1, 2005 from http://www.mentalhealthcommission.gov/.

No Child Left Behind (NCLB). (2002). Act of 2001, Pub. L. No. 107–110, § 115, Stat. 1425.\

Noel, M. (1982). Public school programs for the emotionally disturbed: Overview. In M. Noel & N. Haring (Eds.), *Progress or change: Issues in educating the emotionally disturbed* (Vol. 2, pp. 1–28). Seattle: University of Washington.

O'Connell, M. E., Boat, T., & Warner, K. E. (2009). *Preventing mental, emotional, and behavioral disorders among young people: Progress and possibilities*. Washington, D.C.: National Academies Press.

Perou, R., Bitsko, R. H., Blumberg, S. J., Pastor, P., Ghandour, R. M., Gfroerer, J. C., et al. (2013). Mental health surveillance among children—United States, 2005–2011. *Morbidity and Mortality Weekly Report Surveillance Summary, 62*(Suppl 2), 1–35.

Raines, T. C., Dever, B. V., Kamphaus, R. W., & Roach, A. T. (2012). Universal screening for behavioral and emotional risk: A promising method for reducing disproportionate placement in special education. *The Journal of Negro Education, 81*(3), 283–296.

Rapport, M. D., Denney, C. B., Chung, K. M., & Hustace, K. (2001). Internalizing behavior problems and scholastic achievement in children: Cognitive and behavioral pathways as mediators of outcome. *Journal of Clinical Child Psychology, 30,* 536–551.

Ringel, J. & Sturm, R. (2001). National estimates of mental health utilization and expenditure for children in 1998. *Journal of Behavioral Health Services and Research, 28,* 319–332.

Romer, D. & McIntosh, M. (2005). The roles and perspectives of school mental health professionals in promoting adolescent mental health. In D. L. Evans, E. B. Foa, R. E. Gur, H. Hendin, C. P. O'Brien, M. E. P. Seligman, & B. T. Walsh (Eds.), *Treating and preventing adolescent mental health disorders: What we know and what we don't know* (pp. 598–615). New York: Oxford University Press.

Serwatka, T. S., Deering, S., & Grant, P. (1995). Disproportionate representation of African Americans in emotionally handicapped classes. *Journal of Black Studies, 25*(4), 492–506.

Skiba, R. J., Poloni-Staudinger, L., Simmons, A. B., Feggins-Azziz, L. R., & Chung, C. (2005). Unproven links can poverty explain ethnic disproportionality in special education? *The Journal of Special Education, 39*(3), 130–144.

Skiba, R., Simmons, A., Ritter, S., Kohler, K., Henderson, M., & Wu, T. (2006a). The context of minority disproportionality: Practitioner perspectives on special education referral. *The Teachers College Record, 108*(7), 1424–1459.

Skiba, R. J., Poloni-Staudinger, L., Gallini, S., Simmons, A. B., & Feggins-Azziz, R. (2006b). Disparate access: The disproportionality of African American students with disabilities across educational environments. *Exceptional Children, 72*(4), 411–424.

Skiba, R. J., Simmons, A. B., Ritter, S., Gibb, A. C., Rausch, M. K., Cuadrado, J., & Chung, C. (2008). Achieving equity in special education: History, status, and current challenges. *Exceptional Children, 74*(3), 264–288.

Tilly, W. (2008). The evolution of school psychology to science-based practice: Problem solving and the three-tiered model. *Best Practices in School Psychology V, 1,* 17–36.

Tolan, P. H. & Dodge, K. A. (2005). Children's mental health as a primary care and concern: A system for comprehensive support and service. *American Psychologist,* 60, 601–614.

United States Department of Health and Human Services. (1999). Mental Health: A Report of the Surgeon General. Rockville, MD: U.S. Department of Health and Human Services, Substance abuse, and Mental Health Services Administration, Center for Mental Health Services, National Institutes of Health, National Institute of Mental Health. Retrieved September 1, 2005, from http://www.surgeongeneral.gov/library/mentalhealth/home.html.

United States Public Health Service. (2000). Report of the Surgeon General's Conference on Children's Mental Health: A National Action Agenda, Washington D.C.: Department of Health and Human Services. Retrieved September 1, 2005, from http://www.surgeongeneral.gov/topics/cmh/childreport.htm.

VanDerHeyden, A. M., Witt, J. C., & Naquin, G. (2003). Development and validation of a process for screening referrals to special education. *School Psychology Review, 32,* 204–227.

Wagner, M., Kutash, K., Duchnowski, A. J., Epstein, M. H., & Sumi, W. C. (2005). The children and youth we serve A national picture of the characteristics of students with emotional disturbances receiving special education. *Journal of Emotional and Behavioral Disorders, 13*(2), 79–96.

Walker, H. M., Colvin, G., & Ramsey, E. (1995). *Antisocial behavior in school: Strategies and best practices*. Pacific Grove: Brooks/Cole.

Walker, H. M., Severson, H., Stiller, B., Williams, G., Haring, N., Shinn, M., & Todis, B. (1988). Systematic screening of pupils in the elementary age range at risk for behavior disorders development and trial testing of a multiple gating model. *Remedial and Special Education, 9*(3), 8–20.

Wallace, J. M., Goodkind, S., Wallace, C. M., & Bachman, J. G. (2008). Racial, ethnic, and gender differences in school discipline among U.S. high school students: 1991–2005. *Negro Education Review, 59*(1–2), 47–62.

Wehmeyer, M. L., & Schwartz, M. (2001). Disproportionate representation of males in special education services: Biology, behavior, or bias? *Education and Treatment of Children, 24*(1), 28–45.

Williams, J. R., Ho, M. L., & Grupp-Phelan, J. (2011). The acceptability of mental health screening in a pediatric emergency department. *Pediatric Emergency Care, 27,* 611–615.

Chapter 4
Instrumentation for Mental Health Screening

Evaluating Screening Instruments

Through universal screening, we have the potential to not only identify a greater proportion of individuals with emotional and behavioral problems, but also to do so at an earlier stage, thereby reducing the severity and long-term impact of the disorder. Moreover, universal emotional and behavioral screening can save time and money by minimizing the number of unnecessary diagnostic tests as well as reducing the length of and need for treatment and hospitalizations. The success of early intervention depends on the accuracy and utility of the method used to identify high-risk children. More research must be done in order to develop screening instruments and to determine whether these instruments have validity of score inferences, are cost-effective, and are linked with beneficial interventions and subsequent outcomes.

When evaluating a screening instrument, researchers first must evaluate the psychometric properties of the measure including norm adequacy, reliability, and validity. Validity, as defined by Messick (1995), is "an integrated judgment of the degree to which empirical evidence and theoretical rationales support the adequacy and appropriateness of inferences and actions based on test scores and other modes of assessment." In assessing the validity of a test, the goal is not to conclude whether the test as an instrument is valid, but rather to assess the degree of validity of specific test scores for making inferences about behavior and subsequent decisions, such as intervention. Thus, validity can be viewed as an accumulation of evidence over time; it is not unlike the general scientific procedures for developing and confirming theories.

When developing a test, the crucial question is the degree to which the test is a valid measure of the construct that we wish to assess, known as construct validity. A construct is a latent or unobservable variable or characteristic of people that we are trying to capture as a test score or scores. The construct of interest in this case is the current behavioral and emotional adjustment of a selected child. Results obtained from the screener, therefore, would inform teachers, school officials, psychologists, and others (e.g., doctors, parents) about a child's behavioral and emotional (or in medical terms "health") status and guide decision-making and intervention accordingly.

M. C. Stiffler, B. V. Dever, *Mental Health Screening at School,* Contemporary Issues in Psychological Assessment, DOI 10.1007/978-3-319-19171-3_4

Two essential steps in determining the usefulness of an instrument are assessing predictive validity, which refers to whether the scores from the screener predict important outcomes of interest, as well as assessing whether the screener can be used to differentiate between groups of children (e.g., those with emotional disorders and those without such problems). By assessing these relationships, we are able to build and expand upon what is known about our proposed construct, thus continuing to accumulate evidence to support the construct validity of a measure.

When the classification of a sample of individuals is known, researchers often use an epidemiological model to determine whether an instrument can correctly classify those people as validity evidence (Derogatis and DellaPietra 1994). In this model, the goal is to maximize the number of true positives and true negatives while minimizing false positives and false negatives. The hit rate is an overall measure of the proportion of cases correctly classified, including both true positives and true negatives. In the case of mental health screening, sensitivity (true positives) indicates the proportion of those individuals with emotional and behavioral problems who are detected by the screener. Specificity (true negatives) indicates the proportion of individuals without emotional and behavioral problems who are identified as such by the screener. When the screener identifies individuals without problems as having problems, this misclassification is referred to as the false positive rate. These types of errors may result in wasted resources and misidentification of children. False negatives occur when the screener does not identify individuals who are having problems, leading to the denial of services to children in need. In screening, false positives are more acceptable than false negatives because it is preferable to identify individuals as needing further assessment when they actually do not, rather than allow individuals to suffer the consequences of mental illnesses without receiving treatment.

One can estimate the predictive power of a screener by determining the positive predictive value (PPV) and negative predictive value (NPV) (see Table 4.1). PPV indicates the proportion of individuals with positive screens who actually have emotional and behavioral problems. A low PPV indicates that a large number of false positives are present. On the other hand, when the PPV is optimized false positives are minimized at the risk of missing true cases. NPV indicates the proportion of patients with negative screens who actually do not have emotional and behavioral problems. When the NPV is low, a large number of false negatives are present.

Table 4.1 Relationships among PPV, NPV, sensitivity, and specificity

	Diagnosed	Not diagnosed	
Positive screen	True positive (a)	False positive (b)	PPV a/a+b
Negative screen	False negative (c)	True negative (d)	NPV d/c+d
	Sensitivity a/a+c	Specificity d/b+d	Overall hit rate a+d/a+d+c+b

PPV Positive predictive value, *NPV* Negative predictive value

One must also keep in mind that the base rate of the outcome of interest will significantly affect the PPV and NPV of a screener (Meehl and Rosen 1955). As Hill et al. (2004) explained, "Sensitivity and specificity of tests may sound impressive when reported without reference to PPV, NPV, and base rates. For example, a test with sensitivity of 0.80 and specificity of 0.95 has a PPV of about 74 % if the base rate is 15 %, but the PPV is reduced to 46 % if the base rate is 5 %" (p. 810). A suggested estimate for an annual base rate of emotional and behavioral problems in a normative elementary school population from high-risk environments would be around 20 % as supported by research (Hill et al. 2004; Campaign for Mental Health Reform 2005; Friedman et al. 1996); however, this base rate will be lower when focusing on a single disorder. Many screening instruments fail to provide PPVs and NPVs, limiting their reporting of findings to sensitivity and specificity.

Bennett and Offord (2001) have suggested that screening methods should have a minimal PPV and sensitivity of 0.50, meaning at least 50 % of the children labeled as high-risk are correctly classified (PPV) and at least half of the children with problems should be detected (sensitivity) in order to justify the use of the screener. Power et al. (1998) considered a cut off score clinically useful if PPV or NPV was greater than or equal to 0.65 and if sensitivity or specificity was approximately 0.50 or greater. Other studies (Carran and Scott 1992; Campbell et al. 2001; Weis et al. 2005), on the other hand, indicated that sensitivity, specificity, PPV, and overall hit rate values should be equal to or greater than 0.80 to support the utility of a screening measure. For the purposes of screening, it seems that a low PPV is more tolerable than a low NPV, as false positives are more acceptable than false negatives at the stage of universal screening. Of course, the higher (closer to 1.0) all of these values are, the better the detection of the instrument. However, in the context of mental health screening, PPV values of at least 0.50 and NPV of at least 0.80 would correspond with the practical purpose of identifying as many children as possible during the screening phase, with a more focused follow-up assessment to help determine which cases were false positives.

The usefulness of a screening measure for identifying children at risk for behavioral, emotional, or academic problems can be assessed by performing a receiver operating characteristic (ROC) curve analysis to evaluate the accuracy of discrimination between children with known problems and those without. The ROC curve is a plot of the true positive rate against the false positive rate when testing different potential cut scores for a diagnostic test (Altman 1991). ROC curves demonstrate the trade-off between sensitivity and specificity: increases in sensitivity are accompanied by decreases in specificity. The area under the ROC curve is a measure of test accuracy. Results from a ROC curve analysis can be used to select an optimal cut score for identifying students at risk for developing emotional and behavioral problems. An area under the curve (AUC) of 1 defines a perfect test, while an area of 0.5 represents a relatively inefficient measure; ROC curve areas of 0.80–0.90 are considered "good" discriminators while 0.90–1 are considered "excellent." Fig. 4.1 presents two ROC curves: the first for an assessment with poor discrimination (AUC = 0.64) and the second for an assessment with excellent discrimination (AUC = 0.99). The green diagonal line represents the scenario for which the

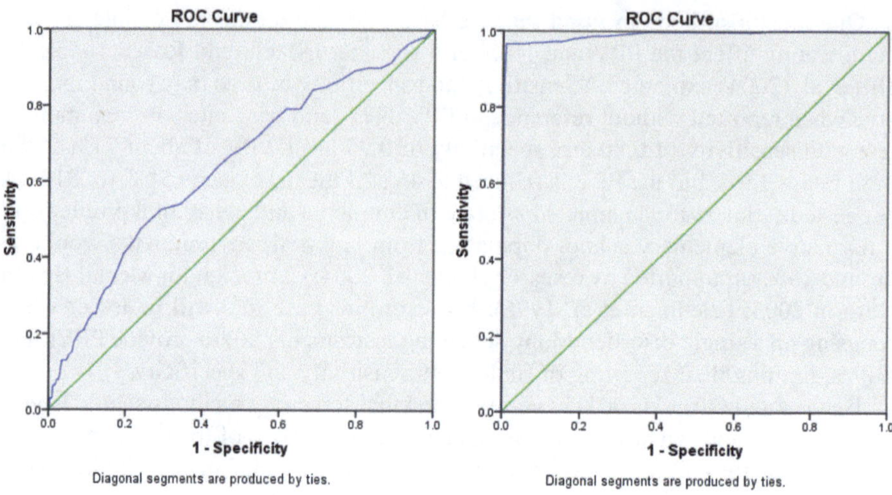

Fig. 4.1 Examples of ROC curve output for the cases of poor *(left)* and excellent *(right)* discrimination

decision to classify or not is no better than chance (0.50). The "height" of the blue curve above the diagonal is an indication of how much better an instrument is at classification as compared with flipping a coin.

Glover and Albers (2007) claimed that when evaluating screening instruments, the user should evaluate their: (a) appropriateness for intended use, (b) psychometric adequacy, and (c) usability. In this chapter, we present information on screening instruments that we hope will be a first step to selecting one to meet the goals specified by a school or district. To address appropriateness, we provide information on broadband screening measures as well as specific, single-disorder measures; the reader should select the appropriate type of instrument depending upon the constructs of interest. Externalizing problems (which may include hyperactivity/inattention), internalizing problems, and difficulties with adaptive skills represent three core constructs that are associated with mental health problems among school-age children (Frick et al. 2009); therefore, in our review we include screeners that assess difficulties in these areas broadly, with a more specific focus on disorders within the domains of externalizing and internalizing. Within each measure, we provide information related to psychometric properties and usability that we hope will assist the reader in selecting a measure with sufficient evidence for its use.

Screening Measures

The following review of child screening measures (see Table 4.2) is meant to be as comprehensive as possible; however, we do not suggest that the review is actually comprehensive as new instruments are being developed on a regular basis.

Table 4.2 Summary of available screening instruments

Instrument type	Instrument	Conditions addressed	Informants and age/grade ranges	# of items	Norming/development sample	[a]Reliability/validity
Broad	Behavioral and Emotional Screening System (BASC-2 BESS)	Psychosocial risk	Parent (Pre-Kindergarten (PK)-12th) teacher (PK-12th) self-report (3rd–12th)	30 items 27 items 30 items	Nationally representative sample of 12,350 children, ages 3 through 18	Adequate reliability and validity; feasible in school settings; PPV ranges from 0.72 to 0.87 across forms and informants in prediction of BSI on BASC-2; NPV ranges from 0.94 to 0.97. Parent form: sensitivity 0.73–0.82 and specificity 0.96–0.97; teacher form: sensitivity 0.80–0.82 and specificity 0.95–0.97; self-report: sensitivity of 0.66, specificity of 0.95

Table 4.2 (continued)

Instrument type	Instrument	Conditions addressed	Informants and age/grade ranges	# of items	Norming/development sample	[a]Reliability/validity
Broad	Pediatric Symptom Checklist (PSC; Jellinek et al. 1986)	Psychosocial risk	Parent (4–16) self-report (11–16)	35 items	206 children, ages 6–12 from three pediatrician's offices—99 % Caucasian, Socioeconomic status (SES) (18 % high, 44 % middle, 38 % low); clinical sample of 31 6–12 year olds, all Caucasian	Adequate reliability and validity; feasible in school settings; No PPV or NPV info provided; parent form: sensitivity from 0.77 to 0.95 and specificity from 0.68 to 1.0; self-report: sensitivity of 0.94, specificity of 0.88 (Jellinek et al. 1995; Simonian and Tarnowski 2001; Murphy et al. 1989; Borowsky et al. 2003)
Broad	Pediatric Symptom Checklist - 17 (PSC-17; Gardner et al. 1999)	Psychosocial risk	Parent (4–16)	17 items	406 children, ages 4–15, recruited from outpatient/inpatient programs, school-based clinics, and physicians; 71 % male	Adequate reliability and validity; adequate sensitivity and specificity at 0.82 and 0.81 respectively; low PPV of 0.15 (Gardner et al. 1999, 2004; Borowsky et al. 2003); more external studies needed

Table 4.2 (continued)

Instrument type	Instrument	Conditions addressed	Informants and age/grade ranges	# of items	Norming/development sample	[a]Reliability/validity
Broad	Strengths and Difficulties Questionnaire (SDQ; Goodman 1997)	Conduct problems, inattention-hyperactivity, emotional symptoms, peer problems, and prosocial behavior as well as a total difficulties score	Parent (4–16), teacher (4–16), and self-report (11–16)	25 items	Originally created in Great Britain, but an American English version has been developed and tested on 9577 children in the US national population sample	Adequate overall reliability and validity; reliability of specific scales is questionable; British version found sensitivity of 0.633, specificity of 0.946. PPV of 0.527, NPV of 0.964 (Goodman and Scott 1999; Mellor 2004; Goodman et al. 2003); need more research on the US version
Broad	Student Risk Screening Scale (SRSS; Drummond 1994)	Behavioral risk	Teacher (K-6; some evidence for extension to K-12)	7 items	Not available	Correlations ranging from 0.61 and 0.68 between SSRS and the SDQ total score (Lane et al. 2007). Internal consistency generally above 0.80 across grade levels; test-retest reliability generally between 0.70 and 0.86 (e.g., Lane et al. 2007, 2008, 2009, 2013; Oakes et al. 2010)

Table 4.2 (continued)

Instrument type	Instrument	Conditions addressed	Informants and age/grade ranges	# of items	Norming/development sample	[a]Reliability/validity
Broad	Systematic Screening for Behavior Disorders (SSBD; Walker and Severson 1992)	Psychosocial risk	Teacher (originally K-6, extended to K-8)	Three stages: 1. Teacher ranking of all students in the classroom, 2. Teacher completion of behavior rating scales for the top three "internalizers" and "externalizers" in the classroom, and 3. Direct observation of those students above the Stage 2 cutoff score using a classroom and playground observational code	454 students and 18 teachers from grades 1–5 in Springfield, or (Walker et al. 1989). Nationally standardized in follow-up work, normative data by age and gender available (Walker and Severson 1992)	Evidence of discriminant validity (externalizing vs. internalizing) and concurrent validity with scales of the CBCL (Walker et al. 1989). Test-retest reliability: 0.83–0.88, internal consistency: 0.82–0.88

Table 4.2 (continued)

Instrument type	Instrument	Conditions addressed	Informants and age/grade ranges	# of items	Norming/development sample	[a]Reliability/validity
Broad	Social, Academic, and Emotional Behavioral Risk Screener (SAEBRS; Kilgus et al. 2013)	Psychosocial risk	Teacher (K-12)	19 items Social: 6 items academic: 6 items emotional: 7 items	Original SABRS was developed based on data from 54 teachers who rated 243 students (K-5) in 3 elementary schools in the Southeastern US about 51 % of the students were white, 33 % were African American, and 10 % were Hispanic/Latino. 20 % of the students received special education services	Adequate reliability and convergent validity; internal consistency of 0.90–0.94. Sensitivity of 0.85–0.97, specificity of 0.73–0.84 (Kilgus et al. 2013)
Specific	Beck Youth Inventories of Emotional and Social Impairment (BYI-II; Beck et al. 2001)	Depression, anxiety, anger, disruptive behavior, and self-concept	Self-report (7–18)	Five 20-item screens	800 children (7–14) stratified based on 1999 census data on, sex, SES and ethnicity; no indication of stratification by geography	Adequate reliability and convergent validity; however discriminant validity evidence is questionable—majority of scales seem to measure same construct (Bose-Deakins and Floyd 2004)

Table 4.2 (continued)

Instrument type	Instrument	Conditions addressed	Informants and age/grade ranges	# of items	Norming/development sample	[a]Reliability/validity
Specific	DISC (Diagnostic Interview Schedule for Children) Predictive Scales (DPS—4.32; Leung et al. 2005)	18 DSM disorders	Self-report (8–18) parent (8–18)	18 scales (total of 98 items) 14 scales (total of 92 items)	Original: 1286 subjects, ages 9–17, from 4 sites (Atlanta, New Haven, New York, and Puerto Rico)	Adequate reliability and validity; sensitivity of 0.68, specificity of 0.91, PPV of 0.34, NPV of 0.98 (Lucas et al. 2001; Leung et al. 2005); need more external validity studies
Specific	Conners 3rd edition (Conners 1973, 2008; Conners et al. 1998)	Oppositional, cognitive problems, hyperactivity	Parent (6–18) and teacher (6–18) and self-report (8–18)	Long forms: 100–115 items; short forms: 41–45 items; ADHD Index (10 items) DSM-IV symptom checklist (18 items)	A representative sample of children ages 6–18, based on 2000 US census data	Adequate reliability and validity; sensitivity from 0.78 to 0.92, specificity from 0.84 to 0.94, PPV from 0.83 to 0.94, and NPV from.81 to 0.92 (Connors et al. 1998); feasible in school settings; limited psychometric evidence for newest edition currently

Table 4.2 (continued)

Instrument type	Instrument	Conditions addressed	Informants and age/grade ranges	# of items	Norming/development sample	[a]Reliability/validity
Specific	AD/HD Comprehensive Teacher's rating scale – 2nd edition (ACTeRS-2; Ullman et al. 1988, 1997)	ADHD	Teacher (K-8th grade)	24 items	2362 students (k-8), no demographic information provided; separate gender norms available	Insufficient reliability evidence; evidence of discrimination between ADHD and controls, manual lacks validity evidence
Specific	ADHD Rating Scale-IV (ADHD-IV, DuPaul et al. 1998)	ADHD	Teacher (5–18) parent (5–18)	18 items 18 items	National sample of 2000 children ages 4–20 matched to 1990 US. census data	Excellent reliability and validity; however, parent form has low specificity evidence; parent form: sensitivity from 0.83 to 0.84, specificity low at 0.49, PPV from 0.54 to 0.58, and NPV from 0.77 to 0.81; teacher form: sensitivity from 0.63 to 0.72. specificity at 0.86, PPV from 0.78–0.79, and NPV from 0.73 to 0.81 (DuPaul et al. 1998)

Table 4.2 (continued)

Instrument type	Instrument	Conditions addressed	Informants and age/grade ranges	# of items	Norming/development sample	[a]Reliability/validity
Specific	Eyberg Child Behavior Inventory; (Eyberg and Pincus 1999)	Conduct problems	Parent (2–16)	36 items	Restandardized in 1999 with 798 children representative of the population in southeastern US on gender, age, ethnicity, SES	Adequate reliability and validity; sensitivity from 0.63 to 0.96, specificity from 0.87 to >0.90, PPV from 0.63 to 0.88 and NPV from 0.82 to 0.96 (Eyberg and Robinson 1983; Boggs et al. 1990; Rich and Eyberg 2001; Weise et al. 2005)
Specific	Sutter-Eyberg Student Behavior Inventory—revised (Eyberg and Pincus 1999)	Conduct problems	Teacher (2–16)	38 items	Problematic norms; 415 elementary school children from 11 schools in Gainesville, FL rated by 52 teachers	Some preliminary reliability and validity evidence; no reliability or validity evidence for older children; need further research

Table 4.2 (continued)

Instrument type	Instrument	Conditions addressed	Informants and age/grade ranges	# of items	Norming/development sample	[a]Reliability/validity
Specific	Revised Children's Manifest Anxiety Scale, second edition (RCMAS–2; Reynolds and Richmond 2008)	Anxiety	Self-report (6–19)	49 items short form—10 items	2368 individuals aged 6–19, representative of the US population in terms of gender, ethnicity, and SES; stratified into three age groups: 6–8, 9–15, 15–19	Reliability estimates improved over the original version: 0.92 for total score and ranging from 0.75–0.86 for scale scores. Similar psychometric properties found for children in Singapore (Ang et al. 2011) and Pakistan (Ahmad and Mansoor 2011)
Specific	State-Trait Anxiety Inventory for Children (Spielberger 1973)	Anxiety	Self-report (9–12)	Two 20 item scales	737 male, 814 female 4th, 5th, and 6th grade elementary school children from six different schools; normative info provided in manual	Self-report: adequate reliability and validity (Carey et al. 1994; Southam-Gerow et al. 2003); unable to differentiate between disorders

Table 4.2 (continued)

Instrument type	Instrument	Conditions addressed	Informants and age/grade ranges	# of items	Norming/development sample	[a]Reliability/validity
Specific	Multidimensional anxiety scale for children, second edition (March 2013)	Anxiety	Self-report (8–19) Parent (8–19)	50 items 50 items	Self-report normative sample includes 1800 children aged 8–19 years. The MASC 2–parent normative sample includes 1600 with an equal number of boys and girls being rated within the 8–19 age range by parents. All normative data is representative of the US and Canadian population in terms of ethnicity/race, gender, and age	Internal consistency 0.92 for self-report, 0.89 for parent-report. Test-retest reliabilities from 0.80 to 0.94 over 1–4 weeks. Studies on original MASC yielded adequate composite reliability—some subscales lower, and initial validity (March et al. 1997); more studies needed to assess discriminant validity; short form has low reliability and lacks validity evidence; limited information on new MASC-2 release to-date beyond information in the manual

Table 4.2 (continued)

Instrument type	Instrument	Conditions addressed	Informants and age/grade ranges	# of items	Norming/development sample	[a]Reliability/validity
Specific	Reynolds Child Depression Scale, second edition (RCDS-2; Reynolds 2010) Reynolds Adolescent Depression Scale, second edition (RADS-2; Reynolds 2002)	Depression	RCDS-2: Self-report (7–13) RADS-2: Self-report (11–20)	30 items short form—11 items	RCDS-2: A new standardization sample of students, drawn from 11 states, stratified closely to match the US census data for gender and ethnic background. The new sample also included children in Grade 2. RADS-2: Sample of 3300 adolescents, stratified to match 2000 US census data.	RCDS-2: Internal consistency coefficients range from 0.87 to 0.91. RADS-2: Internal consistency coefficients range from 0.80 to 0.94. Four factors identified as dysphoric mood, anhedonia-negative affect, negative self-evaluation, and somatic complaints. These factors have been upheld in independent analyses (Osman et al. 2010)
Specific	Children's Depression Inventory 2 (CDI 2; Kovacs 2010)	Depression	Parent (7–17) teacher (7–17) self-report (7–17)	Parent: 17 items teacher:12 items self-report: 28 items self-report short form: 12 items	1100 children aged 7–17 years from 26 different states in the US; stratified by ethnicity, age, gender; 600 teachers, 800 parents; also includes clinical sample	Acceptable reliability and classification accuracy with total score values of: Sensitivity at 0.83, specificity of 0.73, PPV 0.76, and NPV of 0.81

Table 4.2 (continued)

Instrument type	Instrument	Conditions addressed	Informants and age/grade ranges	# of items	Norming/development sample	[a]Reliability/validity
Specific	Center for Epidemiological Studies Depression Scale Modified for Children (CES-DC; Faulstich et al. 1986)	Depression	Self-report (6–17)	20 items	Adapted from adult CES-D which was validated on three samples in Kansas City, MO (n=1173) Washington County, MD ($n1$=1673, $n2$=1089) using household interview surveys	Poor reliability and validity in children, but better for adolescents (Faulstich et al. 1986). In a recent meta-analysis, average internal consistency was 0.88, average sensitivity was 0.76, and average specificity was 0.71, average PPV values ranged from 0.08 to 0.32, and NPV values ranged from 0.12 to 0.98
Specific	Columbia Depression Scale (CDS; Shaffer et al. 2000)	Depression, suicide	Self-report (11–17)	22 items	Derived by selecting items from the DISC—no norming sample	Lacking reliability and validity evidence (Shaffer et al. 2000)

Table 4.2 (continued)

Instrument type	Instrument	Conditions addressed	Informants and age/grade ranges	# of items	Norming/development sample	[a]Reliability/validity
Specific	Beck scale for suicidal ideation (Beck et al. 1979)	Suicidal risk	Self-report (adolescents and adults)	21 items	178 adults in psychiatric outpatient and inpatient settings—insufficient adolescent sample	No reliability and validity information available for adolescents (Beck et al. 1979)
Specific	Suicidal Ideation Questionnaire Jr. (SIQ-JR), Suicidal Ideation Questionnaire (SIQ), (Reynolds 1988, 1991)	Suicidal risk	Self-report (7–9 grade—SIQ JR; 10–12 grade—SIQ)	SIQ Jr—15 items SIQ—30 items	Convenience 7–9 grade sample of 1290 for SIQ-JR; convenience 10–12 grade sample of 890 for SIQ; from three Midwestern schools; info on gender representation is provided	Adequate reliability; adequate convergent validity; good sensitivity ranging from 0.83 to 1.0; low specificity from 40 to 70%; questionable cut score (Reynolds 1991)
Specific	The suicide risk screen (Eggert et al. 1994)	Suicide ideation, suicide attempts, depression, and substance use	Self-report (14 years and older)	20 items—embedded in the health status questionnaire 2.0	Norms not provided	Adequate reliability and validity; good sensitivity at 0.87 to 1.0, but lower specificity ranging from 0.54 to.64 (Thompson and Eggert 1999)

Table 4.2 (continued)

Instrument type	Instrument	Conditions addressed	Informants and age/grade ranges	# of items	Norming/development sample	[a]Reliability/validity
Specific	Columbia Health/Suicide Screen (CSS; Shaffer et al. 2004)	Depression, suicide	Self-report (11–18)	14 items	Convenience sample of 1729 9th – 12th graders from 7 NY high schools	PPV is low at 12–16 %; NPV 99 %; sensitivity of 0.75 to 0.88 and specificity of 0.83 (Shaffer et al. 2004); more research needed

BESS Behavioral and Emotional Screening System, *PSC* Pediatric Symptom Checklist, *PSC—17* Pediatric Symptom Checklist—17, *SDQ* Strengths and Difficulties Questionnaire, *SRSS* Student Risk Screening Scale, *SSBD* Systematic Screening For Behavior Disorders, *SAEBRS* Social, academic, and emotional behavioral risk screener, *BDI* Beck Youth Inventories of emotional and social impairment, *Conners-3* Conners 3rd edition *DPS—4.32* DISC (Diagnostic Interview Schedule for Children) Predictive Scales, , *ACTeRS-2* AD/HD Comprehensive Teacher's Rating Scale—2nd edition, *ADHD-IV* ADHD Rating Scale-IV, *RCMAS-2* Revised Children's Manifest Anxiety Scale Second Edition, *STAIC* State-Trait Anxiety Inventory for Children, *RCDS-2* Reynolds Child Depression Scale Second Edition, *CDI* 2 Children's Depression Inventory 2, *CES-DC* Center for Epidemiological Studies Depression Scale Modified for Children, *CDS* Columbia Depression Scale, *SIQ-JR* Suicidal Ideation Questionnaire Jr., *SIQ* Suicidal Ideation Questionnaire, *CSS* Columbia Health/Suicide Screen

[a] For screening purposes only—not diagnostic, but rather an indication for further assessment

We focused on those measures specifically developed for elementary school-aged children that had been the subject of research studies and contain information on psychometric properties in their manuals.

Broadband Screening Measures

The existence of brief, broadband screeners may provide an important piece of the infrastructure needed to convince school districts and health care providers that early identification is not only beneficial to children, but also can be practically delivered in schools and primary care settings. Traditionally, the content of emotional and behavioral screeners has been comprised of symptoms of disorders. When using symptom-based assessment to screen for a number of disorders, researchers often must sacrifice brevity and cost effectiveness in order to have broad coverage of symptomatology. Therefore, many symptom-based screeners focus on an individual disorder in order to maximize symptom coverage of that particular disorder. Although screening for symptoms of specific disorders indicates an important step in the acceptance of emotional and behavioral screening in general, this procedure also leads to a failure to identify large numbers of children who may have problems other than the target screening condition. A broadband screening measure would ameliorate this problem by covering a number of problem areas in one brief measure.

Theoretically, a broadband screener is feasible if one invokes modern temperament and neurological theory and their variants (Gray 1987; Rothbart and Bates 1998). Although beyond the scope of this text, there is an emerging consensus that much of the range of psychopathology seen in childhood is a function of the interplay of flawed emotional, behavioral, and attentional control systems. Further support for this point of view is the finding that comorbidity is highly prevalent in child psychopathology (Rutter and Sroufe 2000). Additional support can be found in the numerous factor analytic studies of child behavior rating scales that produce three or four factor solutions (Reynolds and Kamphaus 2004). These theoretical stances and associated factor analytic findings suggest that a screener that adequately assesses emotional, behavioral, and attentional control systems will be predictive of the onset of a variety of forms of psychopathology and other important outcomes.

For example, Leon et al. (1999) conducted a large-scale study of depression screening in a primary care setting. They found that a large number of patients with false positives met diagnostic criteria for other mental disorders, thus indicating the need to take comorbidity into account and screen for general maladjustment rather than one or a limited number of disorders. Although the screener was meant to identify those with depression, it succeeded in identifying patients with other disorders as well due to overlapping symptomatology. As the first step in a multiple-gated system (discussed in Chap. 6), screeners should simply identify those children with elevated symptomatology, leaving diagnosis of specific disorders to the later gates. Broadband screening measures of child behavior and emotional adjustment are rare, and those that do exist are often too long and time-intensive (more than 40 items) to be considered true screeners. Examples would include: the Achenbach Child Behavior Checklist (CBCL; Achenbach and Edelbrock 1987), Behavior Assessment System for Children–2 (BASC-2; Reynolds and Kamphaus 2004), McDermott Adjustment Scales for Children and Adolescents (ASCA; McDermott et al. 1994), Child/Adolescent Psychiatry Screen (CAPS), Swanson, Nolan, and Pelham Rating Scale -Revised (SNAP-IV-R; Swanson and Carlson 1994), and the McCarney Behavior Evaluation Scale—2 (McCarney and Leigh 1990).

Therefore, a need exists for the development of brief, multidisorder child screening measures of emotional and behavioral adjustment. Several of the screening instruments listed below are broad, multidisorder instruments that have potential to serve this need; however, these instruments are nascent, and more information is needed about their psychometric properties across populations and time.

Pediatric Symptom Checklist (PSC)

One measure that may be considered a true, multidisorder screener is the PSC (Jellinek et al. 1986): a parent-report, 35-item symptom list developed from the lengthier Washington Symptom Checklist and used in primary care settings with school-aged children (ages 4–16). This measure has been extensively studied with a range of economically, racially, and clinically diverse samples and has been found to have strong internal consistency, test-retest reliability, interrater agreement, and validity for identifying children who would benefit from further, more intensive assessment (Jellinek et al. 1986, 1995; Jellinek and Murphy 1988; Murphy et al. 1992; Simonian and Tarnowski 2001; Stoppelbein et al. 2005; Walker et al. 1989). It has been found to have good sensitivity, ranging from 0.77 to 0.95, and specificity, ranging from 0.68 to 1.0 (Jellinek et al. 1995; Jellinek and Murphy 1990; Simonian and Tarnowski 2001; Stoppelbein et al. 2005; Walker et al. 1989). Although designed for use in primary care settings, the PSC has also been shown to correlate highly with teacher ratings of child symptomatology and academic failure. The PSC has also identified students whose difficulties were unknown to school staff, thus suggesting that it may be of use in school settings as well (Murphy et al. 1989). However, a teacher version of this instrument does not currently exist.

Pagano et al. (2000) adapted the PSC into self-report format (PSC-Y) and found that this measure correlated highly with teacher and parent ratings of child dysfunction as well as self-reported measures of depression and anxiety. The PSC-Y identified children with internalizing symptoms that were missed by parents, thus supporting the superiority of self-report measures in assessing internalizing symptoms. Gall et al. (2000) found support for the use of the PSC-Y in a high school-based health center environment as well. It demonstrated acceptable levels of sensitivity (0.94) and specificity (0.88) in identifying children at psychosocial risk (Pagano et al. 2000); PPV and NPV were not reported. However, the AUC of the PSC-Y was 0.66, which is lower than the 0.8 needed to be considered satisfactory. Therefore, caution should be used in making classification decisions based on the PSC-Y.

Gardner et al. (1999) created a short form of this instrument, Pediatric Symptom Checklist—17 (PSC-17), which has demonstrated lower preliminary reliability estimates at 0.67 for the total score (Borowsky et al. 2003). This instrument has been found to have adequate sensitivity at 0.82 and specificity at 0.81; however, its PPV was found to be quite low at 0.15 (Gardner et al. 1999). Therefore, the authors warn that a positive screen "is not a diagnosis," but rather a "signal for further examination of the child and family" as should be the case with all screening instruments (Gardner et al. 1999, p. 231).

The Behavioral and Emotional Screening System (BESS)

In 2007, Kamphaus and Reynolds developed the BASC-2 Behavioral and Emotional Screening System (BESS), a multi-informant screening system focused on detecting risk for the development of a disorder, rather than any specific diagnosis. The BESS was developed such that item content would reflect the major constructs of child adjustment as contained within the full BASC-2 rating scales. Factor analyses suggest that the self-report includes the domains of internalizing problems, inattention, school problems, and adaptive skills (Dowdy et al. 2011a), the teacher report includes internalizing problems, externalizing problems, school problems, and adaptive skills (Dever et al. 2012), and the parent report includes internalizing problems, externalizing problems, inattention, and adaptive skills (Dowdy et al. 2011b).

The BASC-2 BESS includes two teacher forms (Preschool for ages 3 through 5, and Child/Adolescent for Grades K through 12), two parent forms (Preschool for ages 3 through 5 and Child/Adolescent for Grades K through 12), and a student self-report form (Grades 3 through 12). All forms contain between 25 and 30 items and take 5–10 minutes to administer. All items are rated on a 4-point scale (i.e., *never, sometimes, often, almost always*). A raw score is created by summing the responses to the problem items and the reverse scores of the adaptive behavior items. The raw score is transformed to a total *T*-score, in which higher scores reflect more problems; 20–60 suggests a "Normal" level of risk, 61–70 suggests "Elevated" risk, and scores of 71 or higher suggest an "Extremely Elevated" level of risk.

Reliability evidence was excellent; all split-half reliability coefficients were greater than 0.90 and test-retest reliabilities ranged from 0.80 to 0.91 (Kamphaus and Reynolds 2007). Preliminary validity evidence is also strong; the manual presents strong correlations with other emotional and behavioral measures, the ability to predict important school outcomes, including academic performance, and adequate ROC curve indices (Kamphaus and Reynolds 2007). Interrater reliability estimates ranged from 0.71 to 0.80 for teachers, and from 0.82 to 0.83 for parents. Dever et al. (2013) provided evidence that the BESS screener can provide useful mental health surveillance information across schools and districts, in addition to the individual data gathered. More research, especially validity studies focusing on different outcomes and diverse samples, must be conducted on these new instruments to adequately assess their validity.

Strengths and Difficulties Questionnaire (SDQ)

The SDQ is a 5 minute behavioral questionnaire containing 25 items that generate scores for Conduct Problems, Inattention-Hyperactivity, Emotional Symptoms, Peer Problems, and Prosocial Behavior as well as a Total Difficulties Score. This screener can be completed by parents or teachers of 4–16-year olds and also includes a self-report version for 11–16-year olds. The SDQ was developed in Great Britain based on theory using Diagnostic and Statistical Manual of Mental Disorders-IV (DSM-IV) (APA 1994) criteria as well as factor analyses. Since its development, the SDQ has been translated into 60 languages and extensively researched worldwide including Great Britain, Australia, Holland, Sweden, Norway, Germany, and Urdu (Becker et al. 2004; Flawes and Dadds 2004; Goodman 2001; Malmberg et al. 2003; Ronning et al. 2004; Van Widenfelt et al. 2003; Vostanis 2006).

In several countries, the total score has been found to have adequate reliability with an internal consistency of 0.76 and test-retest reliability of 0.96; however, the internal consistency of the individual scales, with the exception of the inattention-hyperactivity scale, has been questionable. This is especially true for Peer Problems which has an alpha of 0.51 (Goodman and Scott 1999; Mellor 2004). In 2003, Goodman, Ford, Simmons, Gatward, and Meltzer performed a ROC curve analysis on a British community sample of 7984 5–15 year olds using the SDQ and found a sensitivity of 0.633, specificity of 0.946, PPV of 0.527, and NPV of 0.964. Sensitivity varied by diagnosis with 70 to 90 % of conduct, hyperactivity, depression, developmental disorders, and some anxiety disorders being identified, but only 30–50 % of those children with specific phobias, panic disorders, eating disorders, and separation anxiety being identified. They found that the SDQ, although meant to identify specific disorders, was much better at detecting children with more generalized symptomatology due to the high level of comorbidity as well as the overlap of symptomatology in child psychopathology.

Lane et al. (2012a) provide a chapter summarizing the psychometric properties and use of the SDQ. They highlight the low false positive rate found in studies by Goodman and colleagues, but the higher false negative rate may be concerning in a universal screening program due to the desire to identify as many children who may need supports as possible. In this chapter, the authors provide several examples of schools that have used the SDQ to inform intervention and prevention efforts from preschool through high school. Additional information regarding the feasibility of use of the SDQ at the preschool level is presented in White et al. (2013).

Taken together, this research suggests that the SDQ (and more specifically, the total score) would be best used as an indicator of general maladjustment with a second step being used to detect specific disorders. Additionally, one must also keep in mind that sensitivity is of the utmost importance when initially screening children for emotional and behavioral problems in order to minimize false negatives. False negatives should be minimal for a first gate screening instrument because it is critical to identify as many children with emotional and behavioral problems as possible at this stage. Children with emotional and behavioral problems who are missed at the first gate are not recoverable through later assessment (as discussed further in Chap. 6).

An American version of the SDQ has been developed more recently and preliminary findings are positive (Bourdon et al. 2005). As opposed to the five factor structure found in England, Dickey and Blumberg (2004) found a stable three factor model in a US sample consisting of internalizing problems, externalizing problems, and a positive construal factor consisting of prosocial items. The worldwide interest in the SDQ and extensive research currently being done provides an excellent opportunity for researchers to examine cross-cultural similarities and differences with regard to psychosocial adjustment.

Systematic Screening for Behavior Disorders

Systematic Screening for Behavior Disorders (SSBD; Walker and Severson 1992) is a multiple-gated procedure developed to identify students in elementary school who are at elevated risk for externalizing or internalizing disorders. Since its initial development, the SSBD has been extended to the middle school grades as well (e.g., Caldarella et al. 2008). This screening procedure consists of three stages. At stage 1, teachers are asked to create two "top 10 lists"—one for students with internalizing issues and another for students with externalizing issues. In this procedure, teachers are instructed that no student can appear on both lists. The top three students on each list (6 in total) continue to stage 2. During stage 2, teachers complete two rating scales for each of these six students, which capture both the behaviors of those children and the frequency or intensity of those behaviors. Any students exceeding the normative criteria on these instruments continue to stage 3. At stage 3, the students who were identified at the end of stage 2 are observed by a trained professional (often a behavioral specialist or school psychologist) both in the classroom and on the playground. Data on engagement and social behavior are recorded in order to frame the results of the rating scales and assist with decisions about intervention or referral.

Initial development of the SSBD yielded stability coefficients ranging from 0.83 to 0.88, and internal consistency coefficients ranging from 0.82 to 0.88 (Walker et al. 1988). In addition, Walker et al. (1990) provided criterion validity evidence for the SSBD based on school records of behavior and special education classifications. Finally, there is sufficient evidence of convergent validity with similar measures, including the SSRS (Lane et al. 2009) and the CBCL (Walker et al. 1988).

Student Risk Screening Scale

The Student Risk Screening Scale (SRSS; Drummond 1994) is a 7-item teacher-report instrument designed to detect risk for behavior problems in grades K-6; more recent research has provided evidence that its use can be extended to grades K-12

(Lane et al. 2008). All items are rated on a scale from 0 to 3, for a total possible score of 21. Based on their total scores, students are categorized into three levels of risk: Low (0–3), Moderate (4–8), and High (9–21). Due to its brevity, teachers can complete the assessment for an entire classroom in approximately 15 minutes, making it a practical choice for universal screening via teacher-report. The SRSS is available both in written and electronic forms.

In terms of validity evidence, Lane et al. (2009) compared the SRSS and the SSBD (Walker and Severson 1992) at the Kindergarten through third grade levels. Students in this study were enrolled in seven elementary schools, and were predominantly White (95 %). SRSS scores were used to predict SSBD risk classification. The SRSS performed similarly to the SSBD at identifying externalizing problems, but performed poorly at identifying children with internalizing problems. However, this aligns well with the original purpose of the SRSS to assess for problems related to antisocial behavior. In addition, among a diverse group of elementary school students, Menzies and Lane (2012) found that SRSS scores predicted the number of office disciplinary referrals a child would receive during an academic year.

Among older groups of students, Lane et al. (2007) found correlations ranging from 0.61 and 0.68 between SRSS and the SDQ total score for middle school students. There is evidence of adequate internal consistency, test–retest stability, and predictive validity (using the criteria of grade point averages, office disciplinary referrals, and out of school suspensions) of the SRSS for use among urban middle school students (Lane et al. 2010). There is also evidence supporting the use of the SRSS among high school students (Lane et al. 2008). Internal consistency and test-retest reliability coefficients are similarly high across grade levels (see Table 4.2).

More recent efforts have adapted the SRSS to include items that assess internalizing difficulties as well, yielding the Student Risk Screening Scale for Internalizing and Externalizing Behaviors (SRSS-IE; Lane et al. 2012b). Although the original SSRS-IE included the original 7 items of the SRSS plus an additional 7 internalizing items, initial factor analytic work among over 2000 students in grades K-6 supported the retention of only 5 internalizing items, for an SRSS-IE scale of 12 items in total (Lane et al. 2012). Preliminary convergent validity evidence suggests that the SRSS-IE predicts both SDQ and SSBD scores among this elementary school sample. Furthermore, the development of an 11-item Student Risk Screening Scale for Early Childhood (SRSS-EC; Lane et al. 2015) has shown initial promise for identifying the internalizing and externalizing difficulties of preschool students.

Social, Academic, and Emotional Behavioral Risk Screener

The social, academic, and emotional behavioral risk screener (SAEBRS; Kilgus et al. 2013) is a 19-item teacher-report screening instrument that consists of three domains: social behavior (6 items), academic behavior (6 items), and emotional behavior (7 items). Students are rated on a 4-point Likert-type scale, from 0 (never) to 3 (almost always). The SAEBRS can be completed in less than 3 minutes per student, and is intended for rating students in grades K-12. Users of the SAEBRS are provided with an overall level of risk for each student rated, as well as risk levels within each of the three domains of interest.

Factor analysis work with the original dual factor SABRS 12-item instrument (prior to the addition of the 7 emotional behavior items) supports the structure of one broad factor (Behavior) under which are two narrow factors (social and academic) at both the elementary (Kilgus et al. 2013) and secondary (Kilgus et al. 2015) grade levels. Across grade levels, internal consistency estimates are similarly high (ranging from 0.89 to 0.94). When multiple teachers rate the same high school student, interrater reliability estimates range from 0.35 to 0.51 (Kilgus et al. 2015). Future research is needed to determine how the addition of the emotional behavior items has changed the psychometric properties of the instrument. Also, longitudinal research is necessary to examine the predictive validity of the SAEBRS in regard to important social, emotional, and academic outcomes of interest.

Specific Screeners for Multiple Disorders

Several child emotional and behavioral screeners consist of a number of quick screens for multiple disorders simultaneously. For example, the *Beck Youth Inventories—Second Edition* (BYI-II; Beck et al. 2005) are designed for children ages 7–18 years and consist of five 20-item self-report scales that assess symptoms of depression, anxiety, anger, disruptive behavior, and self-concept. These scales can be used separately or in combination depending on the child's individual needs and time constraints.

The DISC (Diagnostic Interview Schedule for Children) Predictive Scales—version 4.32 (DPS-4.32; Leung et al. 2005) was updated to include work done on the National Institute of Mental Health (NIMH) DISC-IV (Shaffer et al. 2000), reflecting DSM-IV diagnostic criteria. The DPS–4.32 consists of parent (14 scales with total of 92 items) and youth (18 scales with total of 98 items) questionnaires that assess the likelihood of a young person, ages 8–18, having any of 18 disorders. Additionally, the DPS-4.32 provides a separate impairment module indicating the degree to which a behavior is having a negative impact on the individual's social, academic and family life. The items were derived from the full DISC (Schwab-Stone et al. 1996), by identifying those items that were most predictive of specific diagnoses (Lucas et al. 2001).

In the original version (DPS-2.3), the substantial reduction in scale length was not associated with any significant changes in discriminatory power. Lucas et al. (2001) examined the DPS-2.3 classification accuracy for a number of disorders including simple phobia, social phobia, agoraphobia, Obsessive Compulsive Disorder (OCD), Major Depressive Disorder (MDD), attention deficit hyperactivity disorder (ADHD), ODD, and conduct disorder. They found adequate reliabilities, sensitivities ranging from 0.67 to 1.00, specificities from 0.49 to 0.96, PPV from 0.07 to 0.74, and NPV from 0.87 to 1.00. They concluded that the DPS is a valuable tool for determining subjects who do not need further assessment and for speeding up the structured diagnostic interviewing process; however, external validity studies were lacking.

An examination of the psychometric properties of the new parent DPS-4.32 version using a community sample ($N=541$) of Chinese children found adequate reliability as well as adequate specificity (0.91), and NPVs (0.98); however, sensitivity was a bit low at 0.68 and PPV was found to be 0.34. Once again, more research should be done to reinforce these findings on other samples (Leung et al. 2005).

Specific Screeners

Other child emotional and behavioral screeners tend to focus on one or several specific diagnoses or problems. These screeners can be classified as those with a focus on specific externalizing disorders, and those with a focus on specific internalizing disorders or risk for suicide. Below we review some of the available screening instruments in each category.

Externalizing Measures

Externalizing disorders, especially ADHD, have been the focus of numerous screening measures for children. The Conners 3rd Edition (CRS-3; Conners 1973, 2008; Conners et al. 1997) are symptom-based rating scales that are widely used in schools, mental health clinics, residential treatment centers, pediatric offices, juvenile detention facilities, child protective agencies, and outpatient settings to screen for ADHD, learning problems, and conduct problems. The authors have suggested that the Conners-3 may be used as a screening measure as well as a tool for treatment monitoring, a diagnostic aid, and a research instrument. There are three versions—parent (ages 6 through 18), teacher (ages 6 through 18), and adolescent (ages 8 through 18) self-report—all of which also have short (10 minutes) and long (20 minutes) forms available. The long forms are too extensive to be used as screening measures; however, in addition to short forms of the Conners-3, users also have the option of administering a 10-item ADHD index or the brief DSM-IV and Diagnostic and Statistical Manual for Mental Disorders-V (DSM-V) Symptom Scales.

Previous versions of this instrument have been found to have adequate reliability and validity (e.g., Conners' Rating Scales–Revised (CRS-R); Conners et al. 1997), but were criticized for having too low cutoff scores thus inflating prevalence rates. However, classification indices are quite high with sensitivities ranging from 0.78 to 0.92, specificities ranging from 0.84 to 0.94, PPV ranging from 0.83 to 0.94, and NPV ranging from 0.81 to 0.92 depending on informant (parent, teacher, and adolescent) (Conners et al. 1997). To date, the Conners-3 manual is the best source of psychometric information for these scales. Alpha coefficients ranged from 0.84 to 0.97 across subscales and informants, indicated adequate internal consistency. Test-retest reliabilities ranged from 0.71 to 0.98, and values for interrater reliabilities ranged from 0.74 to 0.94 for the parent form and from 0.52 to 0.82 for the teacher form.

The ADHD Comprehensive Teacher's Rating Scale (ACTeRS-2; Ullman et al. 1988, 1997) is a 24-item teacher-rated ADHD screener created using a normative sample of over 3700 children from kindergarten through 8th grade. The instrument produces four subscales: attention, hyperactivity, social skills, and opposition. Although this scale has adequate reliability, it has not been widely researched and contains little supportive data in the manual concerning validity. The manual also lacks specific information regarding the standardization sample. Ullman et al. (2000) found that the ACTeRS could differentiate between children with and without ADHD as well as children with learning disabilities and those with ADHD. Although it has not been validated as a screening measure, the ACTeRS-2 may serve this purpose more effectively since it has been found to discriminate between children with and without ADHD. Research should be done to examine this possibility.

In a study including students from grades K through 5 in the mid-Atlantic US, Erford and Hase (2006) found adequate internal consistency of the ACTeRS-2 subscales (from 0.89 to 0.93); however, factor analyses in this same study supported a two-factor solution rather than the four factors suggested by the authors of the instrument. The 30-day test-retest reliabilities ranged from 0.80 to 0.89. When compared to a diagnosis from a qualified mental health professional, 83 % of those diagnosed as ADHD-inattentive type (sensitivity: 0.77; specificity: 0.88), and 0.86 % of those diagnosed as ADHD-hyperactive/impulsive type (sensitivity: 0.81; specificity: 0.88) were correctly identified.

The ADHD Rating Scale—IV (ADHD-IV; DuPaul et al. 1998) is an 18-item rating scale for children ages 5–18, containing both parent and teacher versions. It is based upon DSM-IV diagnostic criteria and contains inattention and hyperactivity subscales. The ADHD-IV was standardized on a large nationally-representative sample, and the manual provides excellent reliability and validity (content, internal structure, convergent, divergent, and predictive) evidence (DuPaul et al. 1998). The manual also provides different cutoff scores depending on the purpose of the assessment (rule-out/screening vs. diagnosis). Parent ratings have sensitivities of 0.83–0.84, specificities of 0.49, PPV of 0.54–0.58, and NPV of 0.77–0.81. Teacher ratings produce sensitivities of 0.63–0.72, specificities of 0.86, PPV of 0.78–079, and NPV of 0.73–0.81 (DuPaul et al. 1998). In general, the ADHD-IV is a well-developed instrument that could be used to screen school aged children for ADHD; however, Collett et al. (2003) warn users about the risk of misclassifying youth due to suboptimal sensitivity and specificity. Furthermore, the scale has yet to be updated to match DSM-V diagnostic criteria, and the lack of a self-report may be a limitation for certain contexts and applications.

The Eyberg Child Behavior Inventory (ECBI; Eyberg and Pincus 1999) is a parent-rated 36-item questionnaire designed for use in pediatric settings as a quick screen for disruptive behavior in children ages 2–16. The Sutter-Eyberg student behavior inventory–revised (SESBI-R; Eyberg and Pincus 1999) was created during the 1999 revision of the ECBI as a teacher-rated version and consists of 38 items, 13 of which are new to the SESBI and served to replace non-school related items from the ECBI. The standardization of the SESBI-R is problematic; the norming sample consisted of 415 elementary school children from 11 schools in Gainesville, FL but the SESBI-R is supposed to target children ages 2–16 despite being normed on a more narrow aged group of children (Meikamp 2003).

The ECBI has been found to have adequate reliability and concurrent validity (Boggs et al. 1990). The ECBI was also found to discriminate between normal and conduct-problem adolescents (Eyberg and Robinson 1983). Rich and Eyberg (2001) found the ECBI to have excellent classification accuracy in a sample of children ages 3–6 with a sensitivity of 0.96, specificity of 0.87, PPV of 0.88, indicating that 88 % of the children who exceeded the cutoff score were correctly identified, and NPV of 0.96.

Weis et al. (2005) found the ECBI to be useful for screening children for externalizing disorders, but less useful in discriminating between specific behavior problems. When classifying children with specific externalizing behavior problems, sensitivities ranged from 0.63 for the Conduct problem component of the ECBI to 0.77 for the Inattentive component. Specificities were all above 0.90. They found that all components of the ECBI displayed adequate NPV, ranging from 0.82 to 0.94. The ECBI Inattentive and Oppositional components displayed PPV of 0.85 and 0.80 respectively, while the conduct problem component exhibited lower PPV at 0.63. The SESBI-R has some preliminary reliability and validity evidence; however, no reliability or validity evidence exists for older children (Whiston and Bouwkamp 2003). More research is needed on the SESBI-R.

Internalizing Measures

Other measures focus on internalizing symptoms such as anxiety and depression. These include self-report measures for school-aged children and adolescents such as the Reynolds and Richmond Revised Children's Manifest Anxiety Scale, Second Edition (RCMAS-2; Reynolds and Richmond 2008), the State-Trait Anxiety Inventory for Children (STAIC; Spielberger 1973), the Multidimensional Anxiety Scale for Children, Second Edition (MASC-2; March 2013), the Reynolds Child Depression Scale, Second Edition (RCDS-2; Reynolds 2010), and the Children's Depression Inventory-2 (CDI-2; Kovacs 2010).

The STAIC and RCMAS have been found to have good reliability and criterion-related validity. These tests can differentiate between youth with anxiety disorders and those without any disorders; however, findings are mixed on their ability to discriminate among diagnostic groups, especially between internalizing problems such as anxiety and depression (Kamphaus and Frick 2002; Seligman et al. 2004). This may be due to item content and overlap with depression measures such as the CDI. Seligman and Ollendick (1998) found that approximately 21 % of RCMAS items and 25 % of STAIC items overlapped with items on the CDI. Thus, the STAIC and RCMAS may be best used as first gate screeners in a multiple-gate system even though they were not developed and validated for this purpose. More research is needed to examine the utility of these instruments in a screening capacity.

In 2008, an updated second edition of the RCMAS was developed. This edition has an updated standardization sample, improved psychometric properties with improved reliability over the original version, and additional items meant to expand content coverage and reflect changes in the way children now experience anxiety

(Reynolds and Richmond 2008). Internal consistency of the total score was reported as 0.92 with a test–retest reliability of 0.76. The scale consists of four factors: physiological anxiety, worry, social anxiety, and defensiveness; however, the total score has yielded higher reliability estimates than the factor scores, which should be used with caution in the absence of more psychometric testing (Huberty 2012). Additionally, a short form consisting of the first ten items of the full form was added that yields a short form total anxiety score. The manual suggests that this form would be useful when screening large numbers of children.

The MASC-2 (March 2013) is a recently updated multi-rater anxiety measure with 50-item self-report (MASC 2–SR) and parent (MASC 2–P) rating forms developed for youth aged 8–19. The MASC-2 yields a total score and subscale scores for six disorder-specific areas. Internal consistency estimates are good, at 0.92 for the MASC 2-SR total score and 0.89 for the MASC 2-P total score. However, internal consistency estimates are lower for the individual subscales (median 0.79). Test–retest reliabilities for both forms range from 0.80 to 0.94. Inter-rater reliability across the two informant forms ranged from 0.43 to 0.68. It has been suggested that the MASC 2-SR might be especially useful for school-based screening, as it can be administered by teachers in an RtI model (Fraccaro et al. 2015). The original version of the MASC (March et al. 1997) has been found to have adequate reliability, including test–retest reliability (March and Sullivan 1999; Christopher 2001), as well as good convergent and divergent validities (March et al. 1997). Rynn et al. (2006) used the MASC to discriminate between children with generalized anxiety disorder and children with depression. They found the AUC of 0.623 to be in the poor to fair range. When sensitivity was set at 0.80, maximum specificity was found to be 0.34. This instrument has not been validated as a screening instrument in a multiple-gate screening system. To date, there is limited information on the revised MASC-2.

The CDI-2 (Kovacs 2010) is a revision of the original CDI(Kovacs 1992) that includes new items that focus on the core aspects of childhood depression, revised scales, and new norms that are representative of the US population. The CDI-2 is a comprehensive multi-rater assessment of depressive symptoms in youth aged 7–17 years. It consists of a 28-item self-report form that yields a total score, two scale scores (emotional problems and functional problems), and four subscale scores, a short self-report form that contains 12 items and yields a total score, as well as teacher and parent forms. Self-report items are answered on a 3-point scale, whereas parent- and teacher-report items are answered on a 4-point scale. The correlation between the CDI-2 self-report and self-report short-form was found to be 0.95, indicating that the short-form may prove quite useful for efficient screening. The manual reported acceptable reliability and classification accuracy with total score values of: sensitivity of 0.83, specificity of 0.73, PPV 0.76, and NPV of 0.81.

The RCDS-2 (Reynolds 2010) is another self-report measure intended to assess the severity of depressive symptomatology in children ages 7–13. The RCDS-2 retains the 30 items used in the original measure, but presents updated normative data. It also includes a short form consisting of 11 of the most critical items from full form. Internal consistency coefficients are satisfactory, ranging from 0.87 to 0.91. For the original RCDS, sensitivity of 0.73 and specificity of 0.97 are reported

(Reynolds 1989). This measure has strong reliability and validity evidence with the exception of discriminant validity as it correlates highly with anxiety measures (Kamphaus and Frick 2002). It is advertised for use as a large-scale screening instrument. The Reynolds Adolescent Depression Scale-Second Edition (RADS-2; Reynolds 2002) was designed as a self-report form for informants aged 11–20. Internal consistency coefficients range from 0.80 to 0.94. It contains four factors identified as dysphoric mood, anhedonia-negative affect, negative self-evaluation, and somatic complaints. These factors have been upheld in independent analyses (Osman et al. 2010).

The Center for Epidemiological Studies Depression Scale Modified for Children (CES-DC; Faulstich et al. 1986) was adapted from the adult CES-D. Faulstich and colleagues (1986) found that the measure had poor reliability and validity for children. A recent meta-analysis, on the other hand, suggests that the measure has adequate reliability and validity for children and adolescents (Stockings et al. 2015). Across nine studies, the average internal consistency was found to be 0.88, average sensitivity was 0.76, and average specificity was 0.71. However, average PPV values ranged from 0.08 to 0.32, and NPV values ranged from 0.12 to 0.98, indicating the need for further evidence of the use of this tool as a screening instrument among children and adolescents. Another scale, the Columbia Depression Scale (CDS) is a 22-item self-report scale, derived from the major depression section of the diagnostic interview schedule for children DISC (Shaffer et al. 2000); however, this scale is lacking reliability and validity evidence (Table 4.2).

Suicide Measures

The most severe outcome of mental illness is suicide. As mentioned earlier, suicide has emerged as the third leading cause of death in youth ages 15–24. Furthermore, over 90 % of children and adolescents who commit suicide have at least one mental disorder, the most common type being mood disorders (Campaign for Mental Health Reform 2005; Shaffer et al. 2004). As Shaffer et al. (2004, p. 71) reasoned, "If the risk factors for suicide are both identifiable and treatable, screening teens for untreated mood disorders should be an important component of any suicide prevention program."

A number of screening instruments have been developed in order to assess suicidal risk in adolescents including the Beck Scale for Suicidal Ideation (Beck et al. 1979), the Suicide Risk Screen (Eggert et al. 1994), and the Suicidal Ideation Questionnaire (Reynolds 1989), which yielded adequate sensitivity ranging from 0.83 to 1.00 with less than adequate specificity from 0.40 to 0.70 when used in a Midwestern US high school. The Beck Scale for Suicidal Ideation provides no reliability and validity information for adolescents, and therefore should not be used until this information is collected. The Suicide Risk Screen assesses factors found to predict suicide among adolescents 14 years and older: suicidal ideation, suicide attempts, depression, and substance use (Shaffer et al. 2004; Brent et al. 1999). Thompson and Eggert (1999) found the Suicide Risk Screen to have sensitivity ranging from 0.87 to 1.00, but low specificity from 0.54 to 0.64 in a sample of 581 high school youth.

The Columbia Suicide Screen (CSS; Shaffer et al. 2004) is a 14-item self-report questionnaire that assesses the most important risk factors for suicide among youth ages 11–18. These items are embedded within a larger screen of general health and relationship items, the Columbia Health Screen, in order to avoid a focus on suicide. Shaffer et al. (2004) found this instrument to have adequate sensitivity (0.75) in identifying high school students at-risk for suicide; however, they did recommend a second stage of evaluation in order to "reduce the burden of low specificity" even though the specificity of 0.83 is superior to most other instruments (p. 71). The PPV was very low at 0.16 which would result in 84 false positives for every 16 youths correctly identified. In general, most suicide screens are limited to adolescent and adult populations and suffer from low specificity, which may overburden programs with false positives. The benefit of being able to intervene for those true positives prior to a suicide attempt is difficult to argue; however, it is important to understand that most of those identified will be false positives. Thus, this instrument, and most suicide screening instruments in general, should only be used as first gates in a multi-gate system.

As stated earlier, this review of the available screening instruments is far from exhaustive; additionally, a word of caution is in order. Although an exorbitant number of instruments exist, one must be careful to assess each instrument's psychometric properties before choosing to utilize that instrument. Many of the instruments reviewed above, as well as those left unmentioned, still need more research evidence before one can be truly confident in their psychometric properties as screeners for emotional and behavioral adjustment. Additionally, one must remember that these instruments are not diagnostic, but rather should be used as indicators for further assessment. Finally, issues of diversity and representativeness of the standardization sample must be considered. We revisit this issue in Chapter 8 when we discuss the future of screening research.

References

Achenbach, T. M., & Edelbrock, C. (1987). *Manual for the child behavior checklist and revised child behavior profile*. Burlington: University of Vermont Department of Psychiatry.

Ahmad, R., & Mansoor, I. (2011). What I think and feel: Translation and adaptation of revised children's manifest anxiety scale, second edition (RCMAS-2) and its reliability assessment. *The International Journal of Educational and Psychological Assessment, 8,* 1–11.

Altman, D. G. (1991). *Practical statistics for medical research*. London: Chapman and Hall.

American Psychiatric Association. (1994). *Diagnostic and statistical manual of mental disorders* (4th edn.). Washington, DC: Author.

Ang, R. P., Lowe, P. A., & Yusof, N. (2011). An examination of the RCMAS-2 scores across gender, ethnic background, and age in a large Asian school sample. *Psychological Assessment, 23,* 899–910.

Beck, A. T., Kovacs, M., & Weissman, A. (1979). Assessment of suicidal ideation: The scale of suicide ideation. *Journal of Consulting and Clinical Psychology, 47,* 343–352.

Beck, J. S., Beck, A. T., & Jolly, J. (2005). *Beck youth inventories* (2nd ed.). San Antonio: Psychological Corporation.

Becker, A., Woerner, W., Hasselhorn, M., Banaschewski, T., & Rothenberger, A. (2004). Validation of the parent and teacher SDQ in a clinical sample. *European Child and Adolescent Psychiatry, 13*(II):11-II/16.

Bennett, K. J., & Offord, D. R. (2001). Screening for conduct problems: Does the predictive accuracy of conduct disorder symptoms improve with age? *Journal of the American Academy of Child and Adolescent Psychiatry, 40,* 1418–1425.

Boggs, S. R., Eyberg, S., & Reynolds, L. A. (1990). Concurrent validity of the eyberg child behavior inventory. *Journal of Clinical Child Psychology, 19*(1), 75–78.

Borowsky, I. W., Mozayeny, S., & Ireland, M. (2003). Brief psychosocial screening at health supervision and acute care visits. *Pediatrics, 112,* 129–133.

Bose-Deakins, J. E., & Floyd, R. G. (2004). A review of the Beck youth inventories of emotional and social impairment. *Journal of School Psychology, 42*(4), 333–340.

Bourdon, K. H., Goodman, R., Rae, D. S., Simpson, G., & Koretz, D. S. (2005). The strengths and difficulties questionnaire: U.S. normative data and psychometric properties. *Journal of the American Academy of Child and Adolescent Psychiatry, 44,* 557–564.

Brent, D. A., Baugher, M., Bridge, J., Chen, T., & Chiappetta, L. (1999). Age- and sex-related risk factors for adolescent suicide. *Journal of the American Academy of Child and Adolescent Psychiatry, 38,* 1497–1505.

Caldarella, P., Young, E. L., Richardson, M. J., Young, B. J., & Young, K. R. (2008). Validation of the Systematic Screening for Behavior Disorders in middle and junior high school. *Journal of Emotional and Behavioral Disorders, 16*(2), 105–117.

Campaign for Mental Health Reform. (2005). A public health crisis: Children and adolescents with mental disorders. Congressional briefing. www.mhreform.org/kids. Accessed 1 Sept 2005.

Campbell, J. M., Bell, S. K., & Keith, L. K. (2001). Concurrent validity of the Peabody picture vocabulary test—third edition as an intelligence and achievement screener for low SES African American children. *Assessment, 8,* 85–94.

Carran, D. T., & Scott, K. G. (1992). Risk assessment in preschool children: Research implications for the early detection of educational handicaps. *Topics in Early Childhood Special Education, 12,* 196–211.

Carey, M. P., Faulstich, M. E., & Carey, T. C. (1994). Assessment of anxiety in adolescents: Concurrent and factorial validities of the Trait Anxiety scale of Spielberger's State-Trait Anxiety Inventory for Children. *Psychological reports, 75,* 331–338.

Christopher, R. (2001). *Review of the multidimensional anxiety scale for children. Fourteenth mental measurements yearbook.* Lincoln: Buros Institute.

Collett, B. R., Jeneva, L. O., & Myers, K. M. (2003). Ten-year review of rating scales. V: Scales assessing attention-deficit/hyperactivity disorder. *Journal of the American Academy of Child and Adolescent Psychiatry, 42,* 1015–1037.

Conners, C. K. (1973). Rating scales for use in drug studies with children. *Psychopharmacology Bulletin, 9,* 24–29.

Conners, C. K. (2008). *Conners* (3rd ed.,) Manual Multi-Health Systems. North Tonawanda, NY.

Conners, C. K., Parker, J. D. A., Sitarenios, G., & Epstein, J. N. (1997). The revised conners' parent rating scale (CPRS-R): Factor structure, reliability, and criterion validity. *Journal of Abnormal Child Psychology, 26,* 257–268.

Conners, C. K., Sitarenios, G., Parker, J. D., & Epstein, J. N. (1998). The revised Conners' Parent Rating Scale (CPRS-R): factor structure, reliability, and criterion validity. *Journal of abnormal child psychology, 26*(4), 257–268.

Derogatis, L. R., & DellaPietra, L. (1994). Psychological tests in screening for psychiatric disorder. In M. E. Maruish (Ed.), *The use of psychological testing for treatment planning and outcome assessment* (pp. 22–54). New Jersey: Lawrence Erlbaum Associates.

Dever, B. V., Mays, K. L., Kamphaus, R. W., & Dowdy, E. (2012). The factor structure of the BASC-2 behavioral and emotional screening system teacher form, child/adolescent. *Journal of Psychoeducational Assessment, 30*(5), 488–495.

Dickey, W. C., & Blumberg, S. J. (2004). Revisiting the factor structure of the strengths and difficulties questionnaire: United States, 2001. *Journal of the American Academy of Child and Adolescent Psychiatry, 43,* 1159–1167.

Dowdy, E., Twyford, J. M., Chin, J. K., DiStefano, C. A., Kamphaus, R. W., & Mays, K. L. (2011). Factor structure of the BASC–2 behavioral and emotional screening system student form. *Psychological Assessment, 23*(2), 379.

Dowdy, E., Chin, J. K., Twyford, J. M., & Dever, B. V. (2011). A factor analytic investigation of the BASC-2 behavioral and emotional screening system parent form: psychometric properties, practical implications, and future directions. *Journal of School Psychology, 49,* 265–280

Drummond, T. (1994). The Student Risk Screening Scale (SRSS). Grants Pass, OR: Josephine County Mental Health Program.

DuPaul, G. J., Power, T. J., Anastopoulos, A. D., & Reid, R. (1998). *ADHD rating scale—IV: Checklists, norms, and clinical interpretation.* New York: The Guilford Press.

Eggert, L., Thompson, E., & Hering, J. (1994). A measure of adolescent potential for suicide (MAPS): Development and preliminary findings. *Suicide and Life-Threatening Behavior, 24,* 359–381.

Erford, B. T., & Hase, K. (2006). Reliability and validity of scores on the ACTeRS-2. *Measurement and Evaluation in Counseling and Development, 39*(2), 97.

Eyberg, S., & Pincus, D. (1999). *Eyberg child behavior inventory & sutter-eyberg student behavior inventory—Revised.* Psychological Assessment Resources. Odessa: Psychological Assessment Rescources.

Eyberg, S. M., & Robinson, E. A. (1983). Conduct problem behavior: Standardization of a behavioral rating scale with adolescents. *Journal of Clinical Child Psychology, 12,* 347–354.

Faulstich, M. E., Carey, M. P., Ruggiero, L., Enyart, P., & Gresham, F. (1986). Assessment of depression in childhood and adolescence: An evaluation of the center for epidemiological studies depression scale for children (CES-DC). *American Journal of Psychiatry, 143,* 1024–1026.

Flawes, D. J., & Dadds, M. R. (2004). Australian data and psychometric properties of the strengths and difficulties questionnaire. *Australian and New Zealand Journal of Psychiatry, 38,* 644–651.

Fraccaro, R. L., Stelnicki, A. M., & Nordstokke, D. W. (2015). Review of the Multidimensional Anxiety Scale for Children (2nd ed.). *Canadian Journal of School Psychology, 30,* 70–77.

Frick, P. J., Burns, C., & Kamphaus, R. W. (2009). *Clinical assessment of child and adolescent personality and behavior* (2nd ed.). New York: Springer.

Friedman, R. M., Katz-Leavy, J., Manderscheid, R., & Sondheimer, D. (1996). Prevalence of serious emotional disturbance in children and adolescents. In R. W. Manderscheid & M. A. Sonnenschein (Eds.), *Mental health, United States, 1996* (pp. 71–88). Rockville: Center for Mental Health Services.

Gall, G., Pagano, M. E., Desmond, M. S., Perrin, J. M., & Murphy, J. M. (2000). Utility of Psychosocial Screening at a School-Based Health Center. *Journal of School Health, 70*(7), 292–298.

Gardner, W., Murphy, M., Childs, G., Kelleher, K., Pagano, M., Jellinek, M., McInerny, T. K., Wasserman, R. C., Nutting, P., & Chiappetta, L. (1999). The PSC-17: A brief pediatric symptom checklist including psychosocial problem subscales: A report from PROS and ASPN. *Ambulatory Child Health, 5,* 225–236.

Glover, T. A., & Albers, C. A. (2007). Considerations for evaluating universal screening assessments. *Journal of School Psychology, 45*(2), 117–135.

Goodman R. (1997). The Strengths and Difficulties Questionnaire: A Research Note. *Journal of Child Psychology and Psychiatry, 38,* 581–586.

Goodman, R. (2001). Psychometric properties of the strengths and difficulties questionnaire. *Journal of the American Academy of Child and Adolescent Psychiatry, 40,* 1337–1345.

Goodman, R., & Scott, S. (1999). Comparing the strengths and difficulties questionnaire and the child behavior checklist: Is small beautiful? *Journal of Abnormal Child Psychology, 27,* 17–24.

Goodman, R., Ford, T., Simmons, H., Gatward, R., & Meltzer, H. (2003). Using the strengths and difficulties questionnaire (SDQ) to screen for child psychiatric disorders in a community sample. *International Review of Psychiatry, 15,* 166–172.

Gray, J. (1987). *The psychology of fear and stress.* New York: Cambridge University Press.

Hill, L. G., Lochman, J. E., Coie, J. D., Greenberg, M. T., & The Conduct Problems Prevention Research Group. (2004). Effectiveness of early screening for externalizing problems: Issues of screening accuracy and utility. *Journal of Consulting and Clinical Psychology, 72,* 809–820.

Huberty, T. J. (2012). *Anxiety and depression in children and adolescents: Assessment, intervention, and prevention.* New York: Springer.

Jellinek, M., & Murphy, J. M. (1988). Screening for psychosocial disorders in pediatric practice. *American Journal of Diseases of Children, 109,* 371–378.

Jellinek, M., & Murphy, J. M. (1990). The recognition of psychosocial disorders in pediatric office practice: The current status of the pediatric symptom checklist. *Journal of Developmental and Behavioral Pediatrics, 11,* 273–278.

Jellinek, M. S., Murphy, J. M., & Burns, B. J. (1986). Brief psychosocial screening in outpatient pediatric practice. *The Journal of Pediatrics, 109,* 371–377.

Jellinek, M., Little, M., Murphy, J. M., & Pagano, M. (1995). The pediatric symptom checklist; support for a role in a managed care environment. *Archives of Pediatrics and Adolescent Medicine, 149,* 740–746.

Kamphaus, R. W., & Frick, P. J. (2002). *Clinical assessment of child and adolescent* personality and behavior (2nd ed.). Boston: Allyn & Bacon.

Kamphaus, R. W., & Reynolds, C. R. (2007). *Behavior assessment system for children,* (BASC-2): Behavioral and emotional screening system (BESS) (2nd ed.). Bloomington: Pearson

Kavan, M. G. (1992). *Review of the children's depression inventory. Eleventh mental measurements yearbook.* Lincoln: Buros Institute.

Kilgus, S. P., Chafouleas, S. M., & Riley-Tillman, T. C. (2013). Development and initial validation of the social and academic behavior risk screener for elementary grades. *School Psychology Quarterly, 28*(3), 210–226.

Kilgus, S. P., Sims, W. A., von der Embse, N. P., & Riley-Tillman, T. C. (2015). Confirmation of models for interpretation and use of the social and academic behavior risk screener (SABRS). *School Psychology Quarterly.* http://psycnet.apa.org/psycinfo/2014-40590-001. Accessed 26 June 2015.

Knoff, H. M. (1992). *Review of the children's depression inventory. Eleventh mental measurements yearbook.* Lincoln: Buros Institute.

Kovacs M. (1992). The Children's Depression Inventory (CDI) manual. New York, NY: Multi-Health Systems.

Kovacs, M. (2010). *Children's depression inventory-2.* North Tonawanda: Multi-Health Systems.

Kresanov, K., Tuominen, J., Piha, J., & Almqvist, F. (1998). Validity of child psychiatric screening methods. *European Child and Adolescent Psychiatry, 7,* 85–95.

Lane, K. L., Parks, R. J., Kalberg, J. R., & Carter, E. W. (2007). Systematic screening at the middle school level: Score reliability and validity of the student risk screening scale. *Journal of Emotional and Behavioral Disorders, 15*(4), 209–222.

Lane, K. L., Kalberg, J. R., Parks, R. J., & Carter, E. W. (2008). Student risk screening scale initial evidence for score reliability and validity at the high school level. *Journal of Emotional and Behavioral Disorders, 16*(3), 178–190.

Lane, K. L., Little, M. A., Casey, A. M., Lambert, W., Wehby, J. H., Weisenbach, J. L., et al. (2009). A comparison of systematic screening tools for emotional and behavioral disorders: How do they compare? *Journal of Emotional and Behavioral Disorders, 17,* 93–105.

Lane, K. L., Bruhn, A. L., Eisner, S. L., & Kalberg, J. R. (2010). Score reliability and validity of the student risk screening scale: A psychometrically sound, feasible tool for use in urban middle schools. *Journal of Emotional and Behavioral Disorders, 18,* 211–224.

Lane, K., Menzies, H., Oakes, W., & Kalberg, J. (2012a). *Systematic screenings of behavior to support instruction: From preschool to high school.* New York: Guilford Press.

Lane, K. L., Oakes, W. P., Harris, P. J., Menzies, H. M., Cox, M., & Lambert, W. (2012b). Initial evidence for the reliability and validity of the student risk screening scale for internalizing and externalizing behaviors at the elementary level. *Behavioral Disorders, 37,* 99–122.

Lane, K. L., Oakes, W. P., Ennis, R. P., Cox, M. L., Schatschneider, C., & Lambert, W. (2013). Additional evidence for the reliability and validity of the student risk screening scale at the high school level: A replication and extension. *Journal of Emotional and Behavioral Disorders, 21*, 97–115.

Lane, K. L., Oakes, W. P., Menzies, H. M., Major, R., Allegra, L., Powers, L., & Schatschneider, C. (2015). The student risk screening scale for early childhood: An initial validation study. *Topics in Early Childhood Special Education, 34*(4), 234–249.

Leon, A. C., Kathol, R., Portera, L., Farber, L., Olfson, M., Lowell, K. N., & Sheehan, D. V. (1999). Diagnostic errors of primary care screens for depression and panic disorder. *International Journal of Psychiatry in Medicine, 29*, 1–11.

Leung, P. W. L., Lucas, C. P., Hung, S., Kwong, S., Tang, C., Lee, C., Ho, T., Lieh-Mak, F., & Shaffer, D. (2005). The test-retest reliability and screening efficiency of DISC predictive scales-version 4.32 (DPS-4.32) with Chinese children/youths. *European Child and Adolescent Psychiatry, 14*, 461–465.

Lucas, C. P., Zhang, H., Fisher, P. W., Shaffer, D., Regier, D. A., Narrow, W. E., Bourdon, K., Dulcan, M. K., Canino, G., Rubio-Stipec, M., Lahey, B. B., & Friman, P. (2001). The DISC predictive scales (DPS): Efficiently screening for diagnoses. *Journal of the American Academy of Child and Adolescent Psychiatry, 40*, 443–449.

Malmberg, M., Rydell, A. M., & Smedje, H. (2003). Validity of the Swedish version of the strengths and difficulties questionnaire (SDQ-Swe). *Nordic Journal of Psychiatry, 57*, 357–364.

March, J. S. (2013). *Multidimensional anxiety scale for children* ((MASC-2) 2nd ed.) North Tonawanda: Multi-Health Systems.

March, J. S., Parker, J. D., Sullivan, K., Stallings, P., & Conners, C. K. (1997). The multidimensional anxiety scale for children (MASC): Factor structure, reliability, and validity. *Journal of the American Academy of Child and Adolescent Psychiatry, 36*, 554–565.

March, J. S., Sullivan, K., & Parker, J. (1999). Test-retest reliability of the Multidimensional Anxiety Scale for Children. *Journal of anxiety disorders, 13*(4), 349–358.

Matthey, S., & Petrovski, P. (2002). The children's depression inventory: Error in cutoff scores for screening purposes. *Psychological Assessment, 14*, 146–149.

McCarney, S., & Leigh, J. (1990). *McCarney behavior evaluation scale—2*. Columbia: Educational Services.

McDermott, P., Marston, N., & Stott, D. (1994). *McDermott adjustment scales for children and adolescents*. Phoenix: Ed. And Psych Associates.

Meehl, P. E., & Rosen, A. (1955). Antecedent probability and the efficiency of psychometric signs, patterns, or cutting scores. *Psychological Bulletin, 52*, 194–216.

Meikamp, J. (2003). *[Review of the eyberg child behavior inventory and sutter-eyberg student behavior inventory-revised]. Fifteenth mental measurements yearbook*. Lincoln: Buros Institute.

Mellor, D. (2004). Furthering the use of strengths and difficulties questionnaire: Reliability with younger child respondents. *Psychological Assessment, 16*, 396–401.

Menzies, H. M., & Lane, K. L. (2012). Validity of the student risk screening scale: Evidence of predictive validity in a diverse, suburban elementary setting. *Journal of Emotional and Behavioral Disorders, 20*(2), 82–91.

Messick, S. (1995). Validity of psychological assessment: Validation of inferences from persons' responses and performances as scientific inquiry into score meaning. *American Psychologist, 50*, 741–749.

Murphy, J. M., Jellinek, M. S., & Milinsky, S. (1989). The pediatric symptom checklist: Validation in the real world of middle school. *Journal of Pediatric Psychology, 14*, 629–639.

Murphy, J. M., Reede, J., Jellinek, M. S., & Bishop, S. J. (1992). Screening for psychosocial dysfunction in inner-city children: Further validation of the pediatric symptom checklist. *Journal of the American Academy of Child and Adolescent Psychiatry, 31*, 1105–1111.

Oakes, W. P., Wilder, K. S., Lane, K. L., Powers, L., Yokoyama, L. T., O'Hare, M. E., & Jenkins, A. B. (2010). Psychometric properties of the student risk screening scale: An effective tool for use in diverse urban elementary schools. *Assessment for Effective Intervention, 35*(4), 231–239.

Osman, A., Gutierrez, P. M., Bagge, C. L., Fang, Q., & Emmerich, A. (2010). Reynolds adolescent depression scale—second edition: A reliable and useful instrument. *Journal of Clinical Psychology, 66*(12), 1324–1345.

Pagano, M. E., Cassidy, L. J., Little, M., Murphy, J. M., & Jellinek, M. S. (2000). Identifying psychosocial dysfunction in school aged children: The pediatric symptom checklist as a self-report measure. *Psychology in the Schools, 37,* 91–106.

Power, T. J., Andrews, T. J., Eiraldi, R. B., Doherty, B. J., Ikeda, M. J., DuPaul, G. J., & Landau, S. (1998). Evaluating attention deficit hyperactivity disorder using multiple informants: The incremental utility of combining teacher with parent reports. *Psychological Assessment, 10,* 250–260.

Reynolds, W. (1988). Suicidal Ideation Questionnaire: Professional Manual. Odessa, FL: Psychological Assessment Resources.

Reynolds, W. M. (1989). *Reynolds child depression scale.* Lutz: Psychological Assessment Resources, Inc.

Reynolds W. M. (2002). *Reynolds adolescent depression scale* (2nd edn.). Lutz: Psychological Assessment Resources, Inc.

Reynolds, W. M. (2010). *Reynolds child depression scale* (2nd edn.). Lutz: Psychological Assessment Resources, Inc.

Reynolds, C. R., & Kamphaus, R. W. (2004). *Behavior assessment system for children (BASC-2)* (2 nd edn.). Circle Pines: Pearson.

Reynolds, C. R., & Richmond, B. O. (1985). *"What I think and feel" reynolds child manifest anxiety scale (RCMAS).* Los Angeles: Western Psychological Services.

Reynolds, C. R., & Richmond, B. O. (2008). *Reynolds child manifest anxiety scale (RCMAS-2)* (2nd edn.) Los Angeles: Western Psychological Services.

Rich, B. A., & Eyberg, S. M. (2001). Accuracy of assessment: The discriminative and predictive power of the eyberg child behavior inventory. *Ambulatory Child Health, 7*(3–4), 249–257.

Ronning, J. A., Handegaard, B. H., Sourander, A., & Morch, W. T. (2004). The strengths and difficulties self-report questionnaire as a screening instrument in Norwegian community samples. *European Child and Adolescent Psychiatry, 13,* 73–82.

Rothbart, M. K., & Bates, J. E. (1998). Temperament. In W. Damon (Series Ed.) & N. Eisenberg (Ed.), *Handbook of child psychology: Vol. 3, Social, emotional, and personality development* (5th edn., pp. 105–176). New York: Wiley.

Rutter, M., & Sroufe, L. A. (2000). Developmental psychopathology: Concepts and challenges. *Development and Psychopathology, 12,* 265–296.

Rynn, M. A., Barber, J. P., Khalid-Khan, S., Siqueland, L., Dembiski, M., McCarthy, K. S., & Gallop, R. (2006). The psychometric properties of the MASC in a pediatric psychiatric sample. *Anxiety Disorders, 20,* 139–157.

Schwab-Stone, M., Shaffer, D., Dulcan, M., Jensen, P., Fisher, P., Bird, H., Goodman, S., Lahey, B., Lichtman, J., Canino, G., Rubio-Stipec, M., & Rae, D. (1996). Criterion validity of the NIMH diagnostic interview schedule for children version 2.3 (DISC-2.3). *Journal of the American Academy of Child and Adolescent Psychiatry, 35,* 878–888.

Seligman, L. D., & Ollendick, T. H. (1998). Comorbidity of anxiety and depression in children and adolescents: An integrative review. *Clinical Child and Family Psychology Review, 1,* 125–144.

Seligman, L. D., Ollendick, T. H., Langley, A. K., & Baldacci, H. B. (2004). The utility of measures of child and adolescent anxiety: A meta-analytic review of the revised children's manifest anxiety scale, the state-trait anxiety inventory for children, and the child behavior checklist. *Journal of Clinical Child and Adolescent Psychology, 33,* 557–565.

Shaffer, D., Fisher, P., Lucas, C., Dulcan, M., & Schwab-Stone, M. (2000). NIMH diagnostic interview scale for children version IV: Description, differences from previous versions, and reliability of some common diagnoses. *Journal of the American Academy of Child and Adolescent Psychiatry, 39,* 28–38.

Shaffer, D., Scott, M., Wilcox, H., Maslow, C., Hicks, R., Lucas, C. P., Garfinkel, R., & Greenwald, S. (2004). The columbia suicide screen: Validity and reliability of a screen for youth suicide and depression. *Journal of the American Academy of Child and Adolescent Psychiatry, 41,* 71–79.

Simonian, S. J., & Tarnowski, K. J. (2001). Utility of the pediatric symptom checklist for behavioral screening of disadvantaged children. *Child Psychiatry and Human Development, 31,* 269–278.

Southam-Gerow, M. A., Flannery-Schroeder, E. C., & Kendall, P. C. (2003). A psychometric evaluation of the parent report form of the State-Trait Anxiety Inventory for Children—Trait Version. *Journal of anxiety disorders, 17*(4), 427–446.

Spielberger, C. D. (1973). *State trait anxiety inventory for children.* Palo Alto: Consulting Psychological Press.

Stockings, E., Degenhardt, L., Lee, Y. Y., Mihalopoulos, C., Liu, A., Hobbs, M., & Patton, G. (2015). Symptom screening scales for detecting major depressive disorder in children and adolescents: A systematic review and meta-analysis of reliability, validity and diagnostic utility. *Journal of Affective Disorders, 174,* 447–463.

Stoppelbein, L., Greening, L., Jordan, S. S., Elkin, T. D., Moll, G., & Pullen, J. (2005). Factor analysis of the pediatric symptom checklist with a chronically ill pediatric population. *Developmental and Behavioral Pediatrics, 26,* 349–355.

Swanson, J., & Carlson, C. L. (1994). DSM-IV rating scale for ADHD and ODD. Unpublished manuscript.

Thompson, E. A., & Eggert, L. L.. (1999). Using the suicide risk screen to identify suicidal adolescents among potential high school dropouts. *Journal of the American Academy of Child and Adolescent Psychiatry, 38,* 1506–1514.

Timbremont, B., Braet, C., & Dreessen, L. (2004). Assessing depression in youth: Relation between the children's depression inventory and a structured interview. *Journal of Clinical Child and Adolescent Psychology, 33,* 149–157.

Ullman, R. K., Sleator, E. K., & Sprague, R. L. (1988). *ADD-H comprehensive teacher's rating scale (ACTeRS).* Champaign: MetriTech, Inc.

Ullman, R. K., Sleator, E. K., & Sprague, R. L. (1997). *ADD-H comprehensive teacher's rating scale (ACTeRS).* Champaign: MetriTech, Inc.

Ullman, R. K., Sleator, E. K., & Sprague, R. L. (2000). ACTeRS Teacher & Parent Forms Manual. Champaign, IL.

Van Widenfelt, B. M., Goedhart, A. W., Treffers, P. D., & Goodman, R. (2003). Dutch version of the strengths and difficulties questionnaire (SDQ). *European Child and Adolescent Psychiatry, 12,* 281–289.

Vostanis, P. (2006). Strengths and difficulties questionnaire: Research and clinical applications. *Current Opinion in Psychiatry, 19,* 367–372.

Walker, H. M., & Severson, H. H. (1992). Systematic screening for behavior disorders (SSBD). Longmont: Sopris West.

Walker, H. M., Severson, H. H., Todis, B. J., Block-Pedego, A. E., Williams, G. J., Haring, N. G., & Barckley, M. (1990). Systematic Screening for Behavior Disorders (SSBD) Further Validation, Replication, and Normative Data. Remedial and Special Education, 11(2), 32–46.

Walker, W. O., LaGrone, R. G., & Atkinson, A. W. (1989). Psychosocial screening in pediatric practice: Identifying high-risk children. *Journal of Developmental and Behavioral Pediatrics, 10,* 134–138.

Weis, R., Lovejoy, M. C., & Lundahl, B. W. (2005). Factor structure and discriminative validity of the eyberg child behavior inventory with young children. *Journal of Psychopathology and Behavioral Assessment, 27,* 269–278.

Whiston, S. C., & Bouwkamp, J. C. (2003). *[Review of the eyberg child behavior inventory and sutter-eyberg student behavior inventory-revised]. Fifteenth mental measurements yearbook.* Lincoln: Buros Institute.

White, J., Connelly, G., Thompson, L., & Wilson, P. (2013). Assessing wellbeing at school entry using the strengths and difficulties questionnaire: Professional perspectives. *Educational Research, 55*(1), 87–98.

References

Chapter 5
Alignment of Mental Health Screening with Response to Intervention Approaches

Introduction

Following the most recent reauthorization of the Individuals with Disabilities Education Act, now called the Individuals with Disabilities Education Improvement Act (IDEIA 2004), the response to intervention (RtI) model has come to the forefront of psychological debate and scrutiny. IDEIA now permits the use of alternative models when assessing and determining special education eligibility, including the use of an RtI approach. The act states that a local education agency "may use a process that determines if the child responds to scientific, research-based intervention as a part of the evaluation procedures."

The No Child Left Behind Act (2002) has also helped to set the stage for an RtI revolution by providing a set of requirements whereby states must implement evidence-based instruction and monitor progress to verify the effectiveness of these programs (Brown-Chidsey and Steege 2005). Additionally, the President's Commission on Excellence in Special Education (2002) called for schools to implement identification and assessment models based on students' responses to evidence-based interventions and monitoring of the level of response.

Although RtI theory and practices are traditionally rooted in the areas of academic problems and learning disability assessment (Fairbanks et al. 2007), these principles are beginning to be applied to other disabilities in the emotional and behavioral domain (Cheney et al. 2008; Gresham 2005). We will begin with a discussion of the general principles of RtI, followed by a more specific discussion as to how these principles might be applied to the practice of screening for emotional and behavioral problems.

M. C. Stiffler, B. V. Dever, *Mental Health Screening at School*, Contemporary Issues in Psychological Assessment, DOI 10.1007/978-3-319-19171-3_5

Principles of Response to Intervention

RtI is a multitiered approach to providing prevention and intervention services to all students within a school, which can be applied to both academic and behavioral outcomes of the students (Brown-Chidsey and Steege 2005; Parisi et al. 2014). Within an RtI framework, those individuals who do not respond to intervention even upon attempts to extend, intensify, and modify the intervention based on data-based decision-making may eventually receive a diagnosis of a disability; however, one of the goals of RtI is to identify and intervene with as many students as possible in order to create an opportunity to prevent difficulties from worsening. Thus, RtI is a prevention-based model that stresses the use of evidence-based intervention practices prior to special education referral, moving away from the "wait to fail" approach often utilized in schools. One must also keep in mind that although RtI is often linked exclusively with assessment and special education decision-making, it also serves as a general education-based tool for monitoring student progress and providing effective instruction and academic interventions.

RtI models typically include (Fairbanks et al. 2007; Harris-Murri et al. 2006; Johnson and Smith 2008) (a) a continuum of evidence-based instruction and interventions available to all students, from universal, high quality, scientifically based general education classroom instruction to highly intensive and individualized interventions; (b) regular school-wide screening of academic performance and behavior to monitor the status and progress of all students; (c) decision points to determine if students are performing significantly below the level of their peers on each indicator assessed; (d) implementation of research-based interventions at all tiers and more intensive or different interventions when students do not improve, as determined through data collected in response to an intervention; (e) on-going progress monitoring of student performance throughout intervention phases; and (f) referral and evaluation for special education services if students are nonresponsive to all attempted interventions. Although we will briefly touch upon each of these components, our main focus will be on the implementation of screening within an RtI approach.

Response to Intervention Models: Tiers and Types

A typical RtI model consists of either three or four tiers, most commonly three tiers, derived from the public health model of prevention (Brown-Chidsey and Steege 2005; Glover and DiPerna 2007; see Fig. 5.1). Tier 1 includes all students and reflects the general education curriculum with regular progress monitoring. Universal screening and prevention mechanisms help to identify risk status and rule out inadequate instruction or behavior management. Tier 2 includes those students who are not responding adequately to Tier 1 instruction and prevention as reflected in universal screening and progress monitoring results, and need more intensive and specific instruction in order to be successful. These students often receive small-

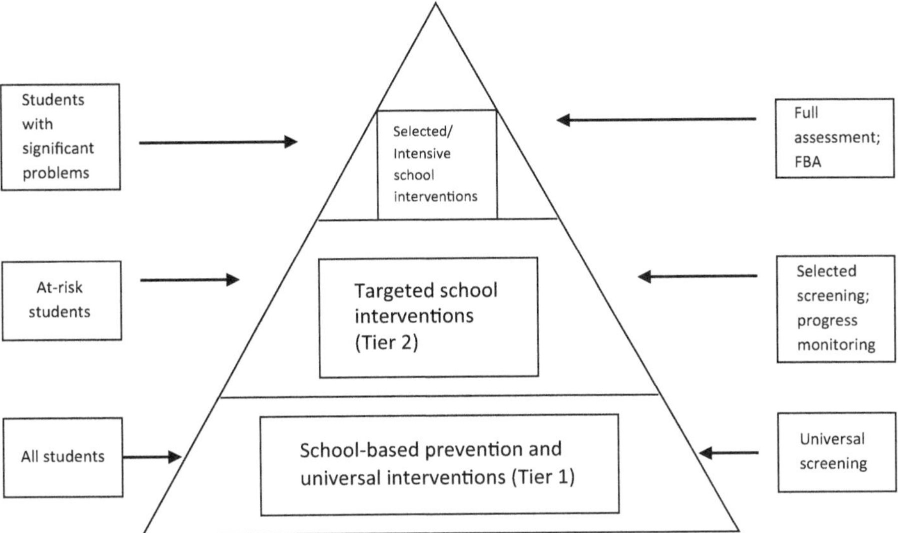

Fig. 5.1 Response to intervention model

group evidence-based instruction for academic problems or short-term, less intensive interventions for behavioral or emotional challenges, along with regular progress monitoring. Tier 3 includes a small subset of students who do not respond to Tier 1 or Tier 2 interventions. This tier necessitates more intensive, individualized interventions and a comprehensive assessment to identify whether the student has a specific disability or meets the criteria for special education. Notably, students do not move from one tier to another without data indicating a need to do so (Brown-Chidsey and Steege 2005).

A four tier model, as described by Klingner and Edwards (2006), might consist of:

Tier 1: Quality instruction within the general education classroom paired with ongoing progress monitoring.

Tier 2: Intensive interventions for those identified using progress monitoring.

Tier 3: Use of a teacher teaming approach, where teams develop interventions for students who continue to display a need for individualized support following the Tier 2 interventions.

Tier 4: Assessment of the severity of the skill deficit, and evaluation of need for special education.

Additionally, two basic versions of RtI exist: the *problem-solving model* and the *standard protocol model*. In the problem-solving model, a four step problem-solving process consisting of problem identification, problem analysis, plan implementation, and problem evaluation is used to select research-based interventions specifically tailored to meet the needs of a particular student. This approach is very sensitive to the unique problems of each individual student, but it is much more difficult to implement and maintain the standardization and controls necessary to evaluate the effectiveness of such an approach. For example, under the problem-solving model, several students with attention difficulties would each have their own individually selected intervention to best match their specific needs and challenges.

The standard protocol model, on the other hand, provides the same empirically validated intervention across all students with similar difficulties. This approach is less individualized, but allows for greater quality control (Atkins 2008). Under the standard protocol model, all students who are identified as having attention difficulties would receive the same intervention, such as teaching them behavioral self-monitoring strategies, and the effectiveness of this approach would be evaluated using progress monitoring across all students. Although this model is not as attentive to the unique needs of every student, it is believed to be more efficient than the problem-solving model both in terms of time and monetary resources needed to learn and delivery the necessary interventions to those students in Tiers 2 and 3.

Applying RtI to Emotional and Behavioral Problems

Gresham (2005) has proposed that RtI be employed as an alternative means to emotional and behavioral disorders (EBD) eligibility determination and in making decisions about modifying or maintaining certain interventions by considering a student's level of responsiveness to a particular intervention. Gresham (2005, p. 331) explained "if a student's behavioral excesses and/or deficits continue at unacceptable levels subsequent to an evidence-based intervention implemented with integrity, then the student can and should be eligible for services." A lack of improvement from the assessed baseline and post-intervention levels of performance might be taken as partial evidence for a need for special education referral. In addition to being used as a tool for identifying children with emotional and behavioral disorders, early screening and identification of all children coupled with the application of RtI and early intervention for those found to be at-risk for emotional and behavioral disorders would lead to more pre-referral intervention in the general-education setting and give the school the ability to act within an intervention framework rather than a "wait to fail" special education eligibility-based framework (Cheney et al. 2008; Gresham 2005).

Universal Screening

Universal screening for behavioral and emotional risk is the initial step to applying the RtI framework to prevention and intervention with behavioral and emotional outcomes in schools. At Tier 1, all students are screened for behavioral and emotional strengths and weaknesses. The purpose of this screening is twofold. First, school leaders and stakeholders review the school-wide results in order to determine whether there is a need to change or supplement the current school-wide prevention strategies being delivered universally. Second, if these Tier prevention programs are deemed to be effective at addressing the behavioral and emotional needs of the majority of the students (typically 80–85 %), then the universal screening data are used to identify those students who should be considered for more targeted interventions at Tier 2.

Parisi et al. (2014) review several common pitfalls to avoid when conducting universal screening within an RtI framework that are applicable to our discussion. First, collecting the data is not enough; screening data must be used in a systematic way to inform decision-making regarding intervention at each tier within RtI. Second, there must be adequate buy-in regarding the importance and use of screening data to make decisions within a narrow timeframe. However, complete consensus is rarely achieved and should not be expected before moving forward with a plan for behavioral RtI. Third, the selection of a screening instrument should not be taken lightly as each instrument will assess only some constructs, utilize certain informants, and need particular resources. We hope our review of some of the more widely-used screening instruments presented in Chapter 4 will assist the reader in the critical task of instrumentation selection.

Finally, those embarking upon an RtI approach to addressing the behavioral and emotional needs of students within their schools should be aware that universal screening is not a one-shot task. Instead, RtI requires an iterative process of assessing the needs of students at all tiers of intervention and making adjustments accordingly. However, there is no single clear answer regarding how frequently universal screening should be conducted at Tier 1. Although, recommendations regarding the frequency of screenings have been put forward, they are largely based on practical concerns rather than data. Most agree that screening should take place at least once a year, usually at the beginning of the school year, in order to determine the course of action for that year (Dowdy et al. 2014; Walker 2010). Others recommend screening three times per academic year, typically in the fall, winter, and spring, in order to inform prevention and intervention decisions (Parisi et al. 2014; Walker et al. 2014). However, there remains a need to empirically evaluate screening frequency recommendations and the stability of screening scores to determine the optimal screening schedule for schools, which may vary depending upon the specific goals of the RtI and the instrumentation used.

Intervention

Gresham (2004) divides behavioral interventions into four broad theoretical categories: (a) applied behavior analysis (ABA) or functional behavioral assessment; (b) social learning theory; (c) cognitive-behavioral therapy; and (d) neobehavioristic stimulus–response (S–R) theory. ABA focuses on identifying the function of the behavior and targeting antecedent and consequent events. A functional behavior analysis (FBA) is a problem-solving process in which broad and specific information about a student's behavior is gathered (e.g., observations, interviews, record review, rating scales, and permanent products) to determine the underlying purpose or function that the behavior serves. This information can then be utilized to develop interventions to change behaviors of concern and to teach new behavior patterns. This may be done by changing antecedent conditions likely to precede the target behavior, teaching alternative prosocial behaviors that serve the same function as the target behavior, and decreasing access to desired consequences that follow the target behavior and increasing access to desired consequences when engaging in appropriate behavior. Social learning theory (Bandura 1977) focuses on the concept of vicarious learning, modeling, and reciprocal determinism, or the effect an individual's behavior has on the environment and vice versa. Cognitive behavioral therapy focuses on changing maladaptive cognitions leading to a change in behavior. Lastly, neobehavioristic S–R models are based on the idea that maladaptive responses are conditioned to stimuli in the environment. Each of these theories makes various assumptions regarding the causes of problem behaviors. Many students require intervention strategies from more than one of these models to be responsive.

In an RtI model, the strength/intensity (i.e., group size, frequency, and duration) of behavioral interventions is organized along a continuum, ranging from Tier 1 classroom interventions to Tier 3 individualized behavior plans. A key concept in RtI is matching the intensity of intervention to the intensity and severity of the presenting problem (Gresham 2004). Additionally, one must keep in mind that simply intensifying an intervention when a child is nonresponsive will not necessarily address the problem if the intervention is not appropriately matched to his or her needs (Daly III et al. 2007). Schools must also balance the strength of the intervention with available resources to ensure that each student is receiving appropriate interventions for his or her skill level. "Not all students will require the most intense form of behavioral or academic interventions and the strength, intensity, and duration of treatment should be increased in direct proportion to the student's unresponsiveness to that treatment" (Gresham 2004, p. 333).

Tier 1, or universal interventions, are meant to target all students in a classroom, school, or district and are delivered to all students in the same manner. Examples of Tier 1 interventions include classroom management strategies, school-wide discipline plans and codes of conduct, district-wide bullying prevention programs, and social skills training in the general education classroom. Universal interventions are estimated to be effective with approximately 80–90 % of a given school population (Colvin et al. 1993; Sugai et al. 2002).

Tier 2, or selected, interventions target those students who are unresponsive to Tier 1 interventions. These students are considered to be at-risk for emotional and behavioral problems and require more targeted interventions often delivered in a small group setting. Tier 2 interventions may include daily behavior report cards, behavioral contracts, self-management strategies, social skills training groups, and token systems. As explained by Gresham (2004, p. 330), "these interventions typically are not based on an analysis of behavioral function but can be characterized more accurately as behavior modification rather than behavior analytic."

Lastly, Tier 3, or targeted, interventions focus on the 1–5 % of the student population that do not respond to Tier 2 interventions, are responsible for 40–50 % of behavioral disruptions in the schools, and drain 50–60% of the school and classroom resources (Colvin et al. 1993; Sugai et al. 2002). These interventions are more intense, individualized, and comprehensive than Tier 1 or Tier 2 interventions. These interventions often use functional behavioral assessment methods to develop individualized behavior plans that may include strategies such as the development of social stories, daily communication with parent, and teaching of positive replacement behaviors.

Progress Monitoring

In order to monitor student progress adequately and make decisions regarding the effectiveness of interventions and student gains, or lack thereof, schools must collect data frequently and evaluate change over time using these data (Cheney et al. 2008). Methods that have been identified as potential progress monitoring tools include behavior ratings scales, permanent products, and systematic direct observation. Although each method offers unique strengths, each also has significant limitations that must be considered when deciding how to effectively monitor progress (Riley-Tillman et al. 2007).

Selecting a behavior rating scale to monitor progress may be appealing due to the ease of use and wide availability of such assessments. However, it is critical to select a scale that adequately covers the domain of interest that is being targeted by the intervention. Most broadband behavior rating scales are not designed to be administered on a frequent basis (e.g., BASC-2, Reynolds and Kamphaus 2004) and narrowband rating scales that have this ability (e.g., ADHD Rating Scale-IV, DuPaul, Power, Anastopoulos, & Reid 1998; BESS, Kamphaus and Reynolds 2007) still include a large number of items, making them somewhat cumbersome to complete repeatedly when the goal is to monitor progress on a bi-weekly, weekly, or even daily basis. Additionally, rating scales tend to lack the sensitivity to detect small daily changes in behavior required for frequent progress monitoring. Currently, two rating scales with particular promise for progress monitoring are the BASC-2 Progress Monitor (Reynolds and Kamphaus 2009) and the web-based progress monitoring tool (Marquez et al. 2013), both of which are between 12–20 items, depending upon the form selected. A full discussion of these tools is beyond the scope of this volume; readers are directed to consult the original citations for further information.

The use of permanent products (e.g., social behavior grades, discipline referrals, or token economy charts) for progress monitoring is popular due to the ease of collection and lack of effort needed on the part of the teacher and others interested in monitoring progress. However, although academic permanent products are generated on a daily basis, it is unlikely that school personnel will have access to a sufficient number of behavioral permanent products to monitor progress of individual students frequently. When the behavior of interest is a lower frequency behavior that would warrant a disciplinary referral or other recorded action, then the use of permanent products might be sufficient; however more minor disruptions such as calling out may not have adequate data readily available in the natural environment (Riley-Tillman et al. 2007). Furthermore, the use of permanent products tends to lend itself to the monitoring of externalizing behaviors; progress monitoring for students with internalizing difficulties will likely need to take another form (e.g., rating scales; Severson et al. 2007).

Systematic direct observation (SDO) is a popular method of progress monitoring (Barnett et al. 2006; Riley-Tillman et al. 2007). Unlike naturalistic observation, during which an observer enters a specific setting (e.g., a classroom) and observes all that occurs with no predetermined set of behaviors in mind, systematic direct observation involves objectively observing specific, operationally-defined behaviors in a carefully selected and specified time and place using standardized procedures. Additionally, scoring and summarizing of data is also standardized and should not vary from one observer to another (Salvia and Ysseldyke 2001). Although this method has the potential to provide valuable information regarding a student's behavioral progress, a major obstacle is the amount of time and resources needed to adequately gain a reliable estimate of a target behavior, especially those behaviors of low frequency (Riley-Tillman et al. 2007). Hintze and Matthews (2004) found that up to four observations per day over 4 weeks may be necessary to obtain a reliable estimate of a behavior such as "being on task." Also, similar to permanent products, SDO is often more appropriate for monitoring progress when externalizing behaviors are being targeted, as internalizing problems are more difficult to observe directly.

An alternative and/or supplementary source of information that may be utilized in monitoring behavior is the daily behavior report card (DBRC; Chafouleas et al. 2005), which has been utilized as an intervention and progress monitoring tool and has preliminary support as a supplement to SDO. Typically, a DBRC lists a number of target behaviors on which the student is rated, at least daily, usually by his or her teacher. Riley-Tillman et al. (2007) list four characteristics of a systematic DBRC: "1) the behavior of interest is operationally defined, 2) the observations should be conducted under standardized procedures to ensure consistency in data collection, 3) the DBRC should be used in a specific time and place, and 4) the data must be scored and summarized in a consistent manner" (p. 79). Similar decisions regarding intervention responsiveness were found to be made based on either teacher-based DBRCs or SDO data, providing some evidence for the validity of inferences made based on the DBRC (Riley-Tillman et al. 2007). However, limitations include the influence of rater perception of student behavior and a lower sensitivity to change than a full SDO.

Assessing Responsiveness

One of the central issues associated with RtI concerns how to ascertain whether a student is "adequately" or "inadequately" responding to an intervention following a positive at-risk screen. The development and application of data-based decision criteria to school-wide screening and progress monitoring of at-risk students is needed (Glover and DiPerna 2007). Gresham (2005) recommends that "this decision must be made at the local and individual level by an assessment and placement team and will most certainly vary across cases and schools…" (p. 332). According to Gresham (2005), factors that might affect a student's response to an intervention include the severity and chronicity of the behavior, generalizability of behavior change, treatment strength and integrity, and treatment effectiveness. So how might one assess whether or not an intervention was effective in changing a behavior? Four possible approaches to making this decision include: (1) visual inspection of data, (2) reliable changes in behavior, (3) changes in social impact measures, and (4) social validation (Gresham 2005).

Visual Inspection of Data

Visual inspection of data involves graphing data collected and visually comparing baseline to intervention phases without the use of statistical analyses. One would assume that if a student is responsive to a particular intervention it should be noticeable by simply viewing the data graphically. However, the absence of standards or criteria for deciding what constitutes adequate behavior change may lead to unreliable decision-making.

Reliable Changes in Behavior

In order to ascertain whether a change in behavior is reliable and not due to chance or extraneous variables, five metrics have been proposed (Gresham 2005): (a) absolute level of change indices; (b) reliable change in score indices based on standard error; (c) percent of data points that do not overlap between baseline and intervention phases; (d) percent change between baseline and intervention; and (e) effect size estimates. *Absolute change* examines the amount of behavior change without comparison to other groups. According to this metric, a student is considered "responsive" if the degree of absolute change is large relative to the amount of change between baseline and post-intervention levels of performance, if an individual no longer meets the established criteria for an emotional disturbance, or if behavior problems are completely eliminated (Gresham 2005). One problem with metrics of absolute change is that they do not take functional impairment into account; a student may have a large degree of change between the baseline and post-intervention data, but may still be functionally impaired within the general education setting.

The *reliable change index (RCI)* takes the standard error, or the variability in the distribution of change scores that would be expected if no actual change occurred, of the difference between pre- and post-intervention performance into account. RCI is calculated by subtracting an individual's post-intervention performance on an outcome measure from his/her pre-intervention performance score and dividing by the standard error. Keep in mind that the RCI is affected by the reliability of the outcome measures used. As always, the psychometric properties of the instrument of interest should be considered prior to making decisions based on its results.

To determine the *percentage of nonoverlapping data points (PND)* an individual's baseline scores are plotted against their post-intervention scores and the number of data points from the post-intervention phase that do not overlap with the baseline data points are identified. This number is then divided by the total number of data points in the post-intervention phase (Gresham 2005). Limitations of this metric include: Not reflecting the magnitude of change, and skewed baseline trends (very high or low data points) or outlier data points that affect interpretation. In addition, floor effects can occur when the beginning baseline score is so low that even in the presence of change, no change is reflected in the PND; similarly, ceiling effects can have a detrimental impact on the interpretation of the PND when scores are so high on the measure that absolute change is difficult to detect. In order to avoid some of these potential pitfalls, Gresham (2005) has recommended using the *percentage of change* as an alternative to the PND. This metric compares the mean level of performance during the baseline phase to the mean level of performance during intervention thus minimizing the effect of outliers and floor and ceiling effects. However, a shared limitation of the percent of change is that no clear guidelines exist for determining what magnitude of behavior change is sufficient to say that an individual has responded adequately to the intervention.

As recommended by Gresham (2005), an individual effect size can be calculated without making any assumptions about the distribution of the data points by subtracting the intervention mean from the baseline mean and then dividing this difference by the standard deviation of the baseline mean (Busk and Serlin 1992). A second approach assumes homogeneity of variance in the data points and uses the pooled standard deviation calculated from baseline and intervention phases in the denominator.

Cheney et al. (2008) utilized a daily progress report to monitor the progress of three to five behavioral expectations and the number of class periods a day. At the end of each class period, teachers met briefly with the students to assess their behavioral performance for that period and rated their behavior on a scale of 1–4 on each expectation during that class period. Students were considered "successful" for that day if they earned 75 % of the total points possible. Cheney et al. (2008) attempted to use all five metrics in their RtI study. They preferred the percentage of change to the other metrics, as it allowed the researchers to examine responses based on the number of days a student met the criteria in post-intervention versus baseline. They found that, overall, percentage of change and effect size were more sensitive than absolute change in detecting responses to interventions. The RCI metric failed to identify some students as responsive who actually appeared to be on a positive trajectory, which is problematic for a progress monitoring metric. Furthermore, the PND suffered in performance due to ceiling effects. Although this study recommends using percentage of change, more research on these and other potential metrics of progress monitoring are necessary to effectively implement this phase of an RtI approach to addressing behavioral and emotional problems.

Changes on Social Impact Measures

In addition to assessing the statistical or empirical magnitude of change, it is perhaps even more critical to assess whether progress has translated into perceivable change in the classroom. In other words, change can be statistically significant without being functionally significant. A social impact measure allows us to look at changes that are recognized as important in everyday life (Kazdin 2003). Social impact measures might include days missed from school, school suspensions, number of fights in the classroom, and disciplinary referrals. One drawback to these types of measures, as described in the previous section, is that they are not particularly sensitive to short-term intervention effects. As Gresham (2005, p. 338) explained, "it is often the case that rather large and sustained changes in behavior are required before these changes are reflected on social impact measures."

When addressing social validity in relation to treatment effectiveness in an RtI model, it is important to focus on the perception of intervention effects by others, such as teachers, in addition to objective measures such as attendance. Gresham and Lopez (1996) suggest using teacher and parent normative behavior rating scales as a means of quantifying the social importance of intervention effects. Additionally, comparing a target student's behavior to one of his non-referred peers through observation could also help estimate the social importance and overall functioning of the student in the classroom. Based on current information, best practice may be to supplement the other statistical metrics reviewed previously with one or more social validation measures, in order to determine whether data from both sources offer the same conclusion when monitoring progress.

An Example

Fairbanks and colleagues (2007) described an RtI standard protocol model to address social behavior concerns in a public elementary school. Tier 1 (universal system) was implemented school wide and consisted of explicitly teaching school-wide expectations, implementing a positive reward system to acknowledge meeting those expectations, and regularly reviewing progress toward school-wide goals. The implementation of evidence-based classroom management strategies would also fit into the Tier 1 system.

Students who were identified by teachers as not being successful under the Tier 1 level of intervention then received more targeted, Tier 2, interventions. These interventions may be implemented in a small group setting during which students develop specific skills that they are lacking. Fairbanks and colleagues (2007) used a "check in and check out" (CICO) or a DBRC at this level of intervention. In this study, the CICO procedure was utilized as an intervention rather than a progress monitoring tool. The CICO program was meant to provide students with "a) increased structure and prompts, b) additional instruction in specific skills, and c) increased regular feedback" (Fairbanks et al. 2007; p. 294). Students could earn a total of 36 points each day based upon their behavior during six, 60-minute time periods throughout the school day. Teachers rated the students at the end of each designated time period on a scale of 0–2 and gave the students feedback in the form of praise or corrective feedback. Additionally, each student with a CICO card tallied up their points at the end of the day and reported it to the class. If the students' cumulative points for that day met a certain criterion, the entire class earned a reward. The criterion was increased several times over the course of the study.

Students who continued to be unsuccessful despite Tier 2 interventions, based upon direct observation data and teacher and counselor nomination, then moved to Tier 3 and received more comprehensive assessments to help with choosing or developing a more personally tailored intervention (Fairbanks et al. 2007). In this particular study, a student was considered unresponsive to intervention if he/she showed little to no improvement in behavior, or an increase in problematic behavior. At this stage, a more formal functional behavioral assessment (FBA) was conducted in order to inform an intervention plan. Following completion of the FBA, a behavior plan was developed for each student that included information about the student's strengths, the target behavior, antecedent variables affecting that behavior, perceived maintaining consequences, and alternative behaviors that might be taught in place of the target behavior.

Although the sample sizes in this study were small and generalizability may therefore be limited, results do suggest that the use of RtI logic with behavior problems appears to be promising. The use of the CICO card was effective in improving the behavior of four students whose problem behaviors were unresponsive to general education classroom management practices. Additionally, for four other students whose behaviors did not improve under the use of these Tier 2 interventions, more individualized function-based Tier 3 interventions were effective in reducing their problem behaviors. Furthermore, teacher reports were positive, indicating that the interventions were easy to implement and improved the overall climate of their classrooms.

Conclusion

The RtI framework appears to be a helpful and relevant way to conceptualize the integration of universal screening, early intervention, and regular progress monitoring within a school- or district-wide system of service delivery. By combining universal screening with RtI principles we allow for proactive identification of children at-risk for emotional and behavioral problems and establish baseline data against which to compare the effects of interventions (Severson and Walker 2002). Through this process, we may avoid the development of more serious mental health difficulties and reduce the need for more intensive and expensive treatments (Gresham 2004). In Chapter 7, we will present another example of a screening system being utilized to implement an RtI-type model for emotional and behavioral problems. We hope that this example will bring to life both the strengths and the challenges of the implementation of such an approach in an authentic context.

References

Atkins, M. E. (2008). Dissertation entitled Response to intervention: Incorporation of an increasing intensity design to improve mathematics fluency.

Bandura, A. (1977). *Social learning theory*. Englewood Cliffs: Prentice-Hall.

Barnett, D. W., Elliott, N., Wolsing, L., Bunger, C. E., Haski, H., & McKissick, C., et al. (2006). Response to intervention for young children with extremely challenging behaviors: What it might look like. *School Psychology Review, 35,* 568–582.

Brown-Chidsey, R., & Steege, M. W. (2005). *Response to intervention: Principles and strategies for effective practice*. New York: The Guilford.

Busk, P., & Serlin, R. (1992). Meta-analysis for single-case research. In T. Kratochwill & J. Levin (Eds.), *Single-case design and analysis* (pp. 187–212). Hillsdale: Lawrence Erlbaum.

Chafouleas, S. M., McDougal, J. L., Riley-Tillman, T. C., Panahon, C. J., & Hilt, A. M. (2005). What do daily behavior report cards (DBRCs) measure? An initial comparison of DBRCs with direct observation for off-task behavior. *Psychology in the Schools, 42,* 669–676.

Cheney, D., Flower, A., & Templeton, T. (2008). Applying response to intervention metrics in the social domain for students at risk of developing emotional or behavioral disorders. *The Journal of Special Education, 42,* 108–126.

Colvin, G., Kame'enui, E. J., & Sugai, G. (1993). Schoolwide and classroom management: Reconceptualizing the integration and management of students with behavior problems in general education. *Education and Treatment of Children, 16,* 361–381.

Daly, E. J. III, Martens, B. K., Barnett, D., Witt, J. C., & Olson, S. C. (2007). Varying intervention delivery in response to intervention: Confronting and resolving challenges with measurement, instruction, and intensity. *School Psychology Review, 36,* 562–581.

Dowdy, E., Nylund-Gibson, K., Felix, E., Morovati, D., Carnazzo, K., & Dever, B. V. (2014). Long-term stability of screening for behavioral and emotional risk. *Educational and Psychological Measurement, 74*(3), 453–472. doi:10.1177/0013164413513460.

DuPaul, G. J., Power, T. J., Anastopoulos, A. D., & Reid, R. (1998). *ADHD Rating Scale-IV: Checklists, norms, and clinical interpretation.* New York: Guilford Press.

Fairbanks, S., Sugai, G., Guardino, D., & Lathrop, M. (2007). Response to intervention: Examining classroom behavior support in second grade. *Council for Exceptional Children, 73,* 288–310.

Glover, T. A., & DiPerna, J. C. (2007). Service delivery for response to intervention: Core components and directions for future research. *School Psychology Review, 36,* 526–540.

Gresham, F. M. (2004). Current status and future directions of school-based behavioral interventions. *School Psychology Review, 33,* 326–343.

Gresham, F. M. (2005). Response to intervention: An alternative means of identifying students as emotionally disturbed. *Education and Treatment of Children, 28,* 328–344.

Gresham, F. M., & Lopez, M. F. (1996). Social validation: A unifying concept for school-based consultation research and practice. *School Psychology Quarterly, 11,* 204–227.

Harris-Murri, N., King, K., & Rostenberg, D. (2006). Reducing disproportionate minority representation in special education programs for students with emotional disturbances: Toward a culturally responsive response to intervention model. *Education and Treatment of Children, 29,* 779–799.

Hintze, J. M., & Matthews, W. J. (2004). The generalizability of systematic direct observations across time and setting: A preliminary investigation of the psychometrics of behavioral observations. *School Psychology Review, 33,* 258–270.

Individuals with Disabilities Education Improvement Act. (2004). 20 U.S.C. § 1400.

Johnson, E. S., & Smith, L. (2008). Implementation of response to intervention at middle school: Challenges and potential benefits. *Council for Exceptional Children. Jan-Feb*, 46–52.

Kamphaus, R. W., & Reynolds, C. R. (2007). *Behavior assessment system for children—Second Edition (BASC-2): Behavioral and emotional screening system (BESS)*. Bloomington: Pearson.

Kazdin, A. E. (2003). Clinical Significance: Measuring whether interventions make a difference. In A. E. Kazdin (Ed.), *Methodological issues and strategies in clinical research* (3rd ed., pp. 691–710). Washington D.C.: American Psychological Association.

Klingner, J. K., & Edwards, P. (2006). Cultural considerations with response-to-intervention models. *Reading Research Quarterly, 41,* 108–117.

Marquez, B., Yeaton, P., & Vincent, C. (2013). Behavioral universal screening and progress monitoring with web-based technology. In H. M. Walker & F. M. Gresham (Eds.), *Handbook of evidence-based practices for emotional and behavioral disorders: Applications in schools* (pp. 192–210). New York: Guilford.

No Child Left Behind (NCLB) Act of 2001. (2002). Pub. L. No. 107–110, § 115, Stat. 1425.

Parisi, D. M., Ihlo, T., & Glover, T. A. (2014). Screening within a multitiered early prevention model: Using assessment to inform instruction and promote students' response to intervention. In R. J. Kettler, T. A. Glover, C. A. Albers, & K. A. Feeney-Kettler (Eds.), *Universal screening in educational settings: Evidence-based decision making for schools* (pp.19–46). Washington, DC: American Psychological Association.

President's Commission on Excellence in Special Education. (2002). A new era: Revitalizing special education for children and their families. http://www.ed.gov/inits/commissionsboards/whspecialeducation/reports/pcesefinalreport.pdf. Accessed 16 Sept 2008.

Reynolds, C. R., & Kamphaus, R. W. (2004). *Behavior assessment system for children-Second Edition (BASC-2).* Circle Pines: Pearson.

Reynolds, C. R., & Kamphaus, R. W. (2009). *BASC-2 Progress Monitor.* Minneapolis: NCS Pearson.

Riley-Tillman, T. C., Chafouleas, S. M., & Briesch, A. M. (2007). A school practictioner's guide to using daily behavior report cards to monitor student behavior. *Psychology in the Schools, 44,* 77–89.

Salvia, J., & Ysseldyke, J. E. (2001). *Assessment* (8th ed.). Princeton: Houghton Mifflin.

Severson, H. H., & Walker, H. M. (2002). Proactive approaches for identifying children at risk for sociobehavioral problems. In K. L. Lane, F. M. Gresham, & T. E. O'Shaughnessy (Eds.), *Interventions for Children with or At Risk for Emotional and Behavioral Disorders* (pp. 33–53). Boston: Allyn & Baco

Severson, H. H., Walker, H. M., Hope-Doolittle, J., Kratochwill, T. R., & Gresham, F. M. (2007). Proactive, early screening to detect behaviorally at-risk students: Issues, approaches, emerging innovations, and professional practices. *Journal of School Psychology, 45,* 193–223.

Sugai, G., Horner, R. H., & Gresham, F. M. (2002). Behaviorally effective school environments. In M. Shinn, H. Walker & G. Stoner (Eds.), *Interventions for academic and behavior problems II* (pp. 315–350). Bethesda: National Association of School Psychologists.

Walker, B. A. (2010). Effective schoolwide screening to identify students at risk for social and behavioral Problems. *Intervention in School and Clinic, 46,* 104–110.

Walker, H. M., Small, J. W., Severson, H. H., Seeley, J. R., & Feil, E. G. (2014). Multiple-gating approaches in universal screening within school and community settings. In R. J. Kettler, T. A. Glover, C. A. Albers & K. A. Feeney-Kettler (Eds.), *Universal screening in educational settings: Evidence-based decision making for schools* (pp. 47–75). Washington, DC: American Psychological Association.

Chapter 6
Multiple-Gating and Mental Health Screening

A Multiple-Gated Screening Procedure

Multiple-gated identification procedures are often used when implementing a universal screening program and are generally aligned with acceptable principles of prevention science (Severson et al. 2007; Weisz et al. 2005). A multiple-gated identification procedure begins by screening an entire population for emotional and behavioral difficulties (universal screening). The students identified by the screening instrument as being at-risk for emotional and behavioral problems are then reassessed using a different, often more thorough, assessment tool such as a full behavior rating scale (selected assessment). Lastly, the students who are identified by the second assessment as having emotional or behavioral problems receive a more comprehensive and individual assessment (indicated assessment). In this way, multiple-gating narrows down the population sequentially so as to yield groups of successively more impaired students; as such, decisions about the need for and intensity of intervention will change as a student progresses through each successive gate, as this would indicate a higher need for intervention.

Typically, each successive gate in a multiple-gated system is different in terms of informant, methodology used, or both (Walker et al. 2014). By utilizing multiple approaches and informants, a more comprehensive picture of the child's behavior and emotionality can be drawn, and identification of children with difficulties is not limited by the characteristics of any one informant or approach. This type of procedure should increase identification and diagnostic accuracy as well as reduce costs due to inefficient identification (Hill et al. 2004; Lochman et al. 1995; Walker et al. 2014).

Issues to Consider

Prior to determining the best approach to a multiple-gated system, a number of variables must be considered. One must evaluate the utility of multiple gates, as well as which informants should constitute each gate. In order to be cost-effective

M. C. Stiffler, B. V. Dever, *Mental Health Screening at School*, Contemporary Issues in Psychological Assessment, DOI 10.1007/978-3-319-19171-3_6

and efficient, each gate must account for additional variance in the prediction of difficulties, subsequently narrow down the pool of students who need intervention, and provide additional utility in identifying those true positive cases. Therefore, choices about both the number of gates and number/choice of informants should be guided by available information regarding what each gate and each informant will add to the identification process while simultaneously considering the added costs associated with each new gate.

One could view multiple-informant assessment as a special type of multiple-gate assessment in which different informants constitute the different gates or levels. These two variables are often confounded in research studies, making it difficult to examine the relative utility of each separately; however, these issues must be evaluated separately to discern what combination of gates and informants is most efficient and accurate for a given purpose. Most research studies do not have systematically varied gates and informants in order to examine the relative accuracy of specific gate/informant combinations; rather, they simply have focused on whether a certain multiple-gate procedure was valid in general without testing it against other versions of the procedure (i.e., different informants and number of gates). According to Johnston and Murray (2003), "future research needs to address … the value of different informants at various stages of the assessment process…" (p. 500). Here we review the available information regarding the utility of multiple gates as well as the choice of informants, both within and outside of a multiple-gated framework.

Number of Gates

Currently no consensus exists as to how many levels of assessment, or gates, are optimal for identifying the children in need of mental health services. Commonly, three-gate procedures are employed, as is the case with the Systematic Screening for Behavior Disorders (SSBD; Walker and Severson 1992), which is examined in detail later in this chapter. In contrast, Simonian and Tarnowski (2001) have suggested a two-stage multimethod system of initial identification of risk (i.e., brief and cost-efficient screening) and subsequent diagnostic assessment (i.e., more comprehensive, multimethod battery) of children in pediatric settings with mental health needs. Pagano and colleagues (2000) discussed the implementation of a similar two-stage model in educational settings.

The Conduct Problems Prevention Research Group (Hill et al. 2004; Lochman et al. 1995) has conducted a number of screening procedure studies that included statistical analyses concerning the utility of each informant and gate. Rather than narrowing down the pool of individuals successively at each gate, these studies analyzed whether adding additional screening measures to a regression equation significantly increased classification accuracy. Multiple regression analyses such as these can inform research on multiple-gating procedures; however, they are not truly multiple-gated studies because all data were collected on all students, not just students selected at each successive gate as would be the case in a multiple-gate screening system.

Hill et al. (2004) compared the effectiveness of single versus multiple raters and single versus multiple time-points when screening for externalizing problems. They did not utilize brief instruments designed for the purposes of screening, but rather selected externalizing items from the Teacher Observation of Classroom Adaptation—Revised (TOCA-R; Werthamer-Larsson et al. 1991) and the Child Behavior Checklist (CBCL) and Revised Problem Behavior Checklist (Achenbach 1991). This study compared the predictive validity of six different screening models using logistic regression and Receiver Operating Characteristic (ROC) curve analyses:

1. Teacher kindergarten (K)
2. Teacher 1st grade
3. Teacher K + Teacher 1st
4. Teacher K + Parent K
5. Teacher K + Parent 1st
6. Teacher K + Teacher 1st + Parent K + Parent 1st

They found that single time-point, multiple rater (parent and teacher) screening (Model #4) was the most effective and efficient in predicting externalizing outcomes; however, this study failed to examine the utility of having a parent screener at the first gate, since the teacher report occurred either simultaneously or first in each situation under consideration. Furthermore, none of the conditions implemented a more comprehensive measure at the second gate, since the focus was on assessment at different time-points rather than with different instruments. Due to this focus, the researchers did not have a two-gate, same informant combination because the teacher who rated the child in first grade was a different teacher from the one who rated him or her in kindergarten.

Lochman and the Conduct Problems Prevention Research Group (1995) examined the usefulness of combining two screening measures in screening kindergartners to predict first grade adjustment problems. Like many others who conduct multiple-gating, Lochman and colleagues pulled items from longer measures to create the screening instruments and did not use a more comprehensive measure as the second gate, but rather added an additional informant. This study examined the utility of a multiple-gate procedure consisting of: Gate 1: Teacher screener, Gate 2: Parent screener, and Gate 3: Detailed information about parent practices. Their results indicated that the second gate of the screening procedure (parent ratings) clearly added to the accuracy of the first gate (teacher ratings) in predicting problem behavior; however, adding a third instrument that measured parent practices did not significantly aid in prediction. In this study, one cannot distinguish whether the increase in effective classification was due to the addition of the second gate, a different informant, or both.

A recent study (VanDeventer 2008) utilizing the BASC-2 Behavioral and Emotional Screening System (BESS; Kamphaus and Reynolds 2007) suggested that adding a comprehensive behavior rating scale as a second gate significantly improves identification accuracy. This study examined a subsample of the child (ages

6–11) and adolescent (ages 12–18) Behavior Assessment System for Children—Second Edition (BASC-2; Reynolds and Kamphaus 2004) general population and clinical norm samples (identified by parent report of diagnosis or special education classification) and attempted to address several questions including:

1. Are parents or teachers better as initial informants for screening for mental health problems of childhood?
2. Are two gates better than a single gate?
3. Are different informants better than one informant in a two-gate screening procedure?

The entire sample was screened using the BESS parent and teacher forms. A full BASC-2, parent and teacher version, was utilized as the second gate and given to the sample of children that was identified by the screener at the first gate. Both same informant and different informant procedures were examined. In order to answer the question of one gate versus two gates, the number of false positives before the second gate application was compared to the number of false positives after the second gate application to determine whether adding a second gate increased classification accuracy by significantly decreasing the number of false positives. The number of false negatives created in applying a second gate was also considered. The odds ratio was also examined. If most of the prediction was completed at the first gate then the odds ratio should be quite small; however, if the second gate was needed, then these indices should be greater than one. Results indicated a clinically meaningful improvement in classification accuracy when adding a second gate, either same or different informant, to the first gate screener as evidenced by large decreases in false positives and odds ratios ranging from 2.13 to 10.62 depending on informant combinations. However, research is needed to discern the optimal number of gates for a multiple-gate procedure.

Number of Informants

In child assessment and diagnosis, it is often recommended that ratings be collected from multiple informants including parents, teachers, as well as the youth themselves so as to provide the greatest amount of information possible from which to make decisions (Kamphaus and Frick 2002). In a multiple-gated screening system, we have the opportunity to implement this recommendation across gates or levels of assessment; however, several issues exist when attempting to integrate and interpret ratings from multiple informants.

Agreement Across Informants

When numerous informants indicate a similar problem, then the practitioner can feel more confident in the validity of his or her diagnosis or classification decision;

however, a lack of consistency across ratings from different informants is more often the case, with low agreement among informant ratings from different settings (e.g., parents and teachers, parents and children) and modest agreement among informants from similar settings (e.g., mother and father, two teachers; Achenbach et al. 1987; Grietens et al. 2004; Grills and Ollendick 2003; van der Ende 1999; Youngstrom et al. 2000). In their classic meta-analysis, Achenbach and colleagues (1987) found that the mean correlation between ratings of mothers and fathers was 0.59, between parents and teachers was 0.27, and between children and other informants was only 0.22. This low agreement indicates that informants are not interchangeable, thus suggesting that multiple informant ratings might provide different and useful information (Frick et al. 2009); however, questions still exist regarding why these discrepancies occur as well as what might be the best way to integrate conflicting information.

Several possible explanations may be offered for the low rate of agreement between informants, none of which are mutually exclusive. In fact, it is more likely that a number of these explanations act in unison to produce informant disagreement. As Renk (2005) explains, "Such disagreements may be viewed as bias or error on the part of one of the informants, as support for the variability of children's behavior across situations, as an informant's lack of access to certain types of behavior, as denial of the behavior of interest, or as distortion of information by an informant" (p. 459). In a multiple-gated approach, high agreement among informants might suggest that only one informant (or gate) is necessary and that additional information is not assisting classification accuracy. Although low agreement among informants could indicate the need for multiple informants to gather more useful information about child behavior, it is also important to consider that perhaps more (and different) does not always equate to better prediction (Biederman et al. 1990; Dowdy and Kim 2012).

First, one must consider the possibility that parents, teachers, and children each provide unique and meaningful information. Parents and teachers see the child in different settings and their ratings may reflect true behavior variations across these settings. For example, discrepant inattention ratings between parents and teachers may reflect differences between demands at home and at school. Achenbach and colleagues (1987) provided evidence for the possibility of actual situational variability by showing that informants in different settings show much lower correlations than those in similar settings. If behavior of the child truly varies by setting, such variation is interesting and useful as an indication of actual contextual differences in behavior.

However, one must distinguish whether informants are providing the desired information before concluding that these discrepancies support the value of collecting information from multiple informants. Ratings of child behavior depend on informant characteristics. An informant's impression of another individual is based upon his or her interpretation of that individual's behavior. Thus, all ratings are subject to the characteristics and judgments of the rater. As van der Ende (1999) pointed out, each informant has his or her own personal thresholds about what constitutes problematic behavior, which depend on knowledge of what constitutes normal behavior, expectations of the child, as well as access to a same-aged peer group from which to compare. Teachers have the advantage of observing the child within a peer group thus allowing them to distinguish between maladaptative and normal age-related problem behavior (Schanding and Nowell 2013). Other informant variables that affect ratings include personality characteristics, psychopathology such as depression (Boyle and Pickles 1997; Clarke-Stewart et al. 2003; Youngstrom et al. 2000), and the informant's own motives, biases, and expectations (Grietens et al. 2004; Renk 2005). Additionally, the parent–child relationship has been found to affect parent ratings of child behavior (Clarke-Stewart et al. 2003; Kamphaus and Frick 2002; van der Ende 1999).

Studies have found that agreement between informants varies depending on several factors including the nature of the problem being assessed (Achenbach et al. 1987; Grills and Ollendick 2003; Loeber et al. 1991; Mesman and Koot 2000; Sourander et al. 1999; Youngstrom et al. 2000), the clinical status of the child (Handwerk et al. 1999), the informant's psychological functioning (Youngstrom et al. 2000), and the age of the child (Achenbach et al. 1987; van der Ende 1999). In general, agreement tends to be higher across informants for externalizing problems than for internalizing problems (Achenbach et al. 1987; Grietens et al. 2004; Kolko and Kazdin 1993) and for younger children than for older children (Achenbach et al. 1987; van der Ende 1999).

Which Informant is "Best"?

Clinicians have been found to weigh adult ratings, such as teachers and parents, more heavily for externalizing behaviors, and child self-report more heavily for emotional or internalizing problems (Loeber et al. 1990). Research has supported these decisions, finding that internalizing problems are best identified through self-report (Loeber et al. 1991; Pagano et al. 2000; Smith 2007; Youngstrom et al. 2000), and that children often report fewer externalizing problem behaviors than either parents or teachers. Correlations between child-reported internalizing syndromes and parent- and teacher-reported syndromes have been found to be low to medium at best (Kolko and Kazdin 1993; Mesman and Koot 2000).

Youth self-report of both externalizing and internalizing symptomatology may also become more valuable as the youth gets older since younger children may not have developed the abilities necessary to accurately reflect on and report feelings and behaviors (Grills and Ollendick 2003). Due to cost-effectiveness and efficiency, self-reports have been suggested as a choice for the first gate in a multiple-gated approach among preadolescents and adolescents (Levitt et al. 2007). Sourander and colleagues (1999) found that a community sample of adolescents reported more internalizing and externalizing problems than their parents, including suicidal symptomatology. However, studies involving clinical adolescent samples have found the opposite effect, with parents rating the adolescents' problems as more severe than the adolescents, who tended to minimize problem behavior (Handwerk et al. 1999). Therefore, the clinical status of the adolescent is an important variable to consider when deciding the informants upon which to base diagnostic decisions.

Contradictory opinions exist as to the superiority of parent or teacher ratings. Several studies (Loeber et al. 1991; Youngstrom et al. 2000) have found that teachers reported fewer internalizing and externalizing problems than caregivers or youth; on the other hand, Kaufman et al. (1994) found that teachers identified *more* problems. When comparing parent and teacher ratings to a population-based model, teachers provided estimates of at-risk child behavior that fit this model, whereas parents underreported behavioral and emotional risk (Schanding and Nowell 2013); this suggests that teachers may be a better choice than parents at Gate 1, where false negatives are particularly problematic. Several studies have found mothers to be more accurate in perceiving internalizing problems in children than teachers (Grietens et al. 2004; Loeber et al. 1990; Youngstrom et al. 2000); however, Mesman and Koot (2000) found that teachers were more likely to report internalizing problems than parents. VanDeventer (2008) suggested that the parent BESS screeners were superior to teachers in both the child and adolescent samples. However, the use of the behavioral rating scores might be important to consider; for example, when used to predict achievement, teacher ratings may be more accurate than parent ratings, given the match in context between teacher and school-related outcomes (Juechter et al. 2012).

Wolraich et al. (2004) found that teachers reported higher levels of inattention than parents, perhaps due to differing environmental demands. Reynolds and Kamphaus' (1992) research with teacher rating scales has demonstrated that, on an average, teacher ratings of child behavior are more reliable than parent ratings at preschool, child, and adolescent age levels, and that different teachers rate the same child similarly. Loeber and colleagues (1991) found teacher reports, as compared to child and parent reports, of attention deficit hyperactivity disorder (ADHD) symptoms in elementary school children to be the best predictors of later impairment including suspensions and special education placement. However, Goodman and colleagues (2004) found that teachers and caregivers provided information of roughly equivalent predictive value. Therefore, further research is necessary to help clarify some of these contradictions in informant contributions and accuracy.

Are More Informants Necessarily Better?

Additionally, contradictory opinions exist as to the utility of collecting ratings from multiple informants. Several studies (Biederman et al. 1990; Lochman et al. 1995) found that adding another informant added little variance to the identification process beyond that provided by the first informant. Jones and colleagues (2002) found that the effect of combining parent and teacher ratings was equal to or minimally higher than that of the teacher-only rating. These findings would indicate that multiple informants are not necessary in a multiple-gate screening system, as the costs may outweigh any additional benefit; rather, one could simply have the same informant (e.g., teacher) complete a more comprehensive rating scale for the second gate.

Goodman and colleagues (2003), on the other hand, found that the Strengths and Difficulties Questionnaire (SDQ) best predicted child outcomes when ratings by all possible informants (parents, teachers, and child) were taken into account. Power and colleagues (1998) concluded that a combined informant approach, using both parent and teacher reports, was more successful in predicting the presence of ADHD than the single informant approach. Hill and colleagues (2004) also found parent–teacher models to be superior; however, teacher-only models had good predictive value for both externalizing and delinquency outcomes. Goodman and colleagues (2004) found that SDQ prediction was best when both caregiver and teacher ratings were completed. They also found that self-reports provided little extra information above that provided by either parent or teacher ratings.

VanDeventer (2008) found that utilizing a different informant at the second gate of a two-gate screening system generally improved the accuracy of identifying children and adolescents with emotional and behavioral disorders. The number of false positives decreased significantly when using a different informant as opposed to the same informant as the second gate. These findings would support the use of a different informant for the second gate of a multiple-gate screening system.

In general, the majority of researchers and clinicians continue to emphasize the importance of multi-informant assessment (Jensen et al. 1999; Kamphaus and Frick 2002; Power et al. 1998; Verhulst et al. 1997); however, one must keep in mind that a consensus has not yet been reached on this issue. It is often assumed that more is always better, whether it be number of informants, methods, or levels of assessment; however, this has not always been found to be the case (McFall 2005). Adding scores with lower reliability or validity in identifying students with behavior or emotional difficulties does not increase predictive accuracy, but rather leads to contamination of findings. Furthermore, one reaches a point where adding more measures no longer contributes enough unique variance to be worth the cost in materials, training, and effort. Specific combinations of measures, including different informants and number of gates, must be explored empirically in order to ascertain the most efficient and accurate combination for assessing emotional and behavioral maladjustment. More research is needed to address these complex issues.

Cut Score Selection

Cut score selection depends on the goal and/or purpose for screening. By altering cut scores, sensitivity and specificity may be increased or decreased accordingly. For example, the number of false negatives may be decreased by lowering the cut score; however, this would cause an increase in false positives. The desired balance between these two errors may differ depending on a number of factors including purpose of screening as well as financial and personnel resources. False negative errors result in children with emotional and behavioral problems being missed and denied necessary services; therefore, if the purpose of your measure is to catch all children with emotional and behavioral problems, false negatives should be minimized through the selection of lower cut scores. However, false positives create difficulties in terms of finances, time, and personnel. By serving children who do not necessarily need services, valuable resources are wasted. False positives can also result in unnecessary stress and stigma for the misidentified child and his or her family.

False positives are more acceptable than false negatives for a first gate screening instrument as the goal is typically to catch as many children with emotional and behavioral problems as possible at this stage (Walker et al. 2014). Children with emotional and behavioral problems who are missed at this gate are not recoverable through later assessment and are therefore "lost for good." Hence, most universal screening programs are more tolerant of false positive errors at the first gate, as this limits the number of children who fall through the cracks and miss the opportunity for receiving the necessary intervention. False positive errors can be corrected through the addition of later gates, where those students who may not need additional services can be filtered out using more comprehensive assessments.

For the second gate, false positives and false negatives should be given equal consideration as opposed to the first gate screener where the goal is to minimize false negatives. Positively screened cases at the second gate may be referred for more comprehensive assessment or intensive interventions, requiring more resources and thus making false positives less desirable and more costly. Additionally, false negatives at the second gate would hopefully still be receiving some intervention or monitoring due to being identified at Gate 1. Therefore, cases that were deemed at-risk at Gate 1, but are not identified with problems at Gate 2, can be monitored or followed up appropriately rather than potentially slipping through the cracks as false negatives at the first gate.

As discussed in Chapter 4, performing an ROC curve analysis, comparing children with known problems versus those without, is an important step to understanding the psychometric properties of an instrument. To review, the ROC curve is a plot of the true positive rate against the false positive rate of different possible cut scores for a diagnostic test (Altman 1991). ROC curves demonstrate the trade-off between sensitivity and specificity (increases in sensitivity are accompanied by decreases in specificity) and use the area under the plotted curve as a measure of test accuracy. Results from a ROC curve analysis can be used to select an optimal cut score in the case of developing a new instrument. In addition, a ROC curve analysis can be used to set different cut scores on the same instrument given different purposes, such as initial screening when false negatives should be minimized, and a final gate when false positives should be minimized.

Examples of a Multiple-Gated Approach to Screening

The SSBD (Walker and Severson 1992) is a multiple-gated procedure developed to identify students in elementary school who are at elevated risk for externalizing or internalizing disorders. The SSBD is one of the only multiple-gated procedures found in the literature that is designed to screen for multiple adjustment problems in children as opposed to a single disorder such as ADHD. This screening procedure consists of three stages: (1) teacher ranking of all students in the classroom according to the externalizing and internalizing dimensions; (2) teacher completion of behavior rating scales for the top three "internalizers" and "externalizers" in the classroom, and (3) direct observation of students.

Researchers have found the results of the SSBD procedure to have adequate validity and reliability (see Chapter 4), as well as cost-efficiency, in identifying children in need of services; additionally, the SSBD has been rated favorably by study participants including teachers and psychologists (Philips et al. 1993; Walker et al. 1988; Walker and Severson 1994). However, multiple-gate systems that include teacher training and rankings (i.e., nomination) and classroom observations are relatively expensive in terms of personnel costs as assessed by teachers and other staff time devoted to this task. In addition to the time spent actually completing the task, teachers and observers must also be trained, which increases the costs.

August et al. (1992) utilized a multiple-gated identification system in order to assess for ADHD among 1490 elementary school students. In their procedure, Stage 1 consisted of teachers' ratings of the child's behavior using the Child Behavior Checklist Teacher Report Form (CBCL-TRF) (Achenbach 1991), Stage 2 consisted of parents' ratings using the parent version of the CBCL (Achenbach 1991), and Stage 3 involved the administration of a structured psychiatric interview, the Diagnostic Interview for Children and Adolescents Revised—Parent version (DICA-R-P; Reich and Welner 1990). When the child obtained a T-score of 60 or greater on the Attention Problems scale on the CBCL-TRF, then a CBCL was administered to a parent or guardian. If a T-score of 65 or greater was obtained on the Attention Problems scale of the parent form, then the DICA-R-P was administered at Stage 3 of the assessment. The procedure resulted in an excellent positive predictive value (PPV) with 90% of the children identified in Stage 2 subsequently receiving an ADHD diagnosis at Stage 3, thus suggesting that the three-stage screening procedure maximized the use of time necessary to diagnose ADHD (August et al. 1992). However, the length of the rating scales used in this study is of great concern, especially if this procedure was to be implemented on a large scale.

August et al. (1995) also employed a multiple-gate screening procedure to identify children at-risk for conduct disorder. Once again, they employed a three-gate procedure; however, they chose to utilize a specific section of the Conners Rating Scale in this study. Gate 1 consisted of teachers completing the 10-item Hyperactivity Index of the Revised Conners Teacher Rating Scale for the entire population (CTRS-R; Goyette et al. 1978). In Gate 2, parents of those children who received a score of 1.6 or higher, completed the 10-item Hyperactivity Index of the Revised Conners Parent Rating Scale (CPRS-R; Goyette et al. 1978). Lastly, a set of 15 items was given to assess parent behavioral management practices. It was found that the procedure adequately discriminated children with higher adjustment from those with lower adjustment with all measures contributing significantly to prediction of a child's self-concept, problem behaviors, and social skills (August et al. 1995). Additionally, the procedure predicted diagnostic ratings of psychiatric symptomatology with Gate 1 predicting both ADHD and oppositional defiant disorder (ODD) while Gate 2 added to the prediction of ADHD, but not ODD. Gate 3 contributed to the prediction of ODD, but not ADHD. Thus, it appears that the addition of gates and informants aided in accurate identification of children with behavioral and emotional maladjustment, depending upon the diagnosis of interest.

Although these latter two studies contribute to our knowledge of the use and utility of multiple-gating procedures, they are also limited to a focus on externalizing symptomatology. Furthermore, both studies selected subscales and items from longer measures, rather than using an assessment tool that was designed for the purposes of universal screening. Both studies illustrate the potential of using a second informant at Gate 2; however, this may not be necessary if a different, more comprehensive measure could be completed by the same informant at Gate 2. As both studies used teacher report at Gate 1 and parent report at Gate 2, it is unclear whether similar results would be obtained with different informants (e.g., self-report), utilizing these informants in reverse order, or collecting information from the same informant at both gates.

Conclusions

As with much of the work in universal screening for behavioral and emotional risk, much more research is needed regarding the most effective approach to multiple-gating when seeking to identify students with behavioral and emotional difficulties. Given the goal of universal screening at Gate 1, it makes good sense to choose an assessment that may err on the side of identifying false positives instead of false negatives, in order to avoid allowing students who may need intervention from slipping through the cracks. Due to the aim for universal screening to overidentify, a multiple-gated approach is often necessary from a cost-efficiency perspective as all students who are first identified may not truly need intervention services. However, the questions of optimal number of gates, which informants to use, and what methodology to use at each gate have yet to be answered and may depend largely on the purpose and goals of the implementers of the screening program. Although youth self-report is often the easiest and cheapest to gather, youth may be best at reporting their own internalizing behavior, particularly in middle school and beyond. When interested in externalizing issues, research suggests that teachers and/or parents are the informants of choice. Although these are good rules of thumb that are grounded in preliminary research, more work is needed to disentangle the contributions of multiple gates, multiple methods, and multiple informants and examine the best approach to move from universal screening to diagnostic or indicated assessment within a multiple-gating framework (Fig. 6.1).

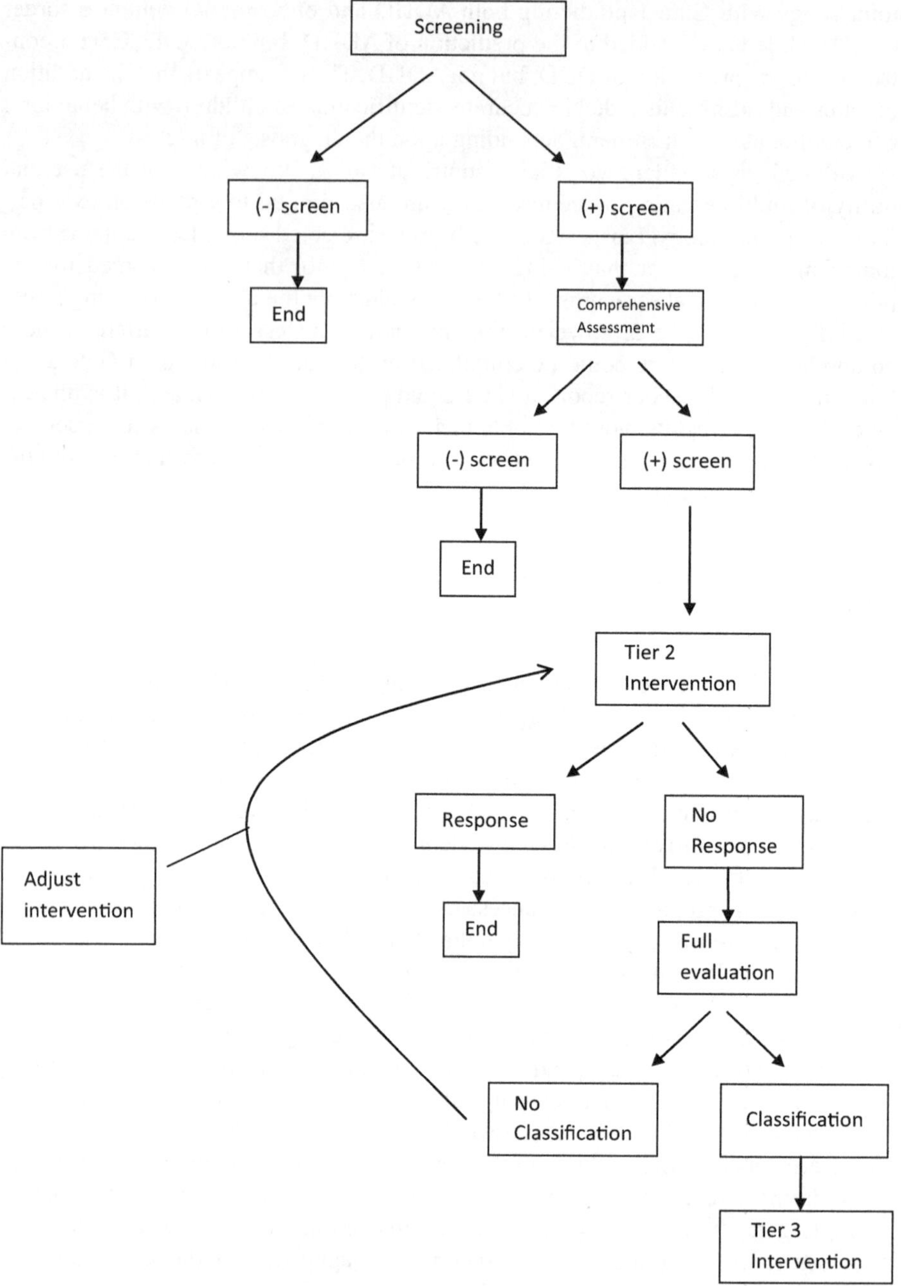

Fig. 6.1 Flow chart for universal screening in a public health model of service delivery

References

Achenbach, T. M. (1991). *Integrative guide to the 1991 CBCL/4–18, YSR, and TRF Profiles*. Burlington: University of Vermont.

Achenbach, T. M., McConaughy, S. H., & Howell, C. T. (1987). Child/adolescent behavioral and emotional problems: Implications of cross-informant correlations for situational specificity. *Psychological Bulletin, 101,* 213–232.

Altman, D. G. (1991). *Practical statistics for medical research*. London: Chapman and Hall.

August, G. J., Ostrander, R., & Bloomquist, M. J. (1992). Attention deficit hyperactivity disorder: Epidemiological screening method. *American Journal of Orthopsychiatrics, 62,* 387–396.

August, G. J., Realmuto, G. M., Crosby, R. D., & MacDonald, A. W. (1995). Community-based multiple-gate screening of children at risk for conduct disorder. *Journal of Abnormal Child Psychology, 23,* 521–544.

Biederman, J., Keenan, K., & Faraone, S. V. (1990). Parent-based diagnosis of attention deficit disorder predicts a diagnosis based on teacher report. *Journal of the American Academy of Child and Adolescent Psychiatry, 29,* 698–701.

Boyle, M. H., & Pickles, A. R. (1997). Influence of maternal depressive symptoms on ratings of childhood behavior. *Journal of Abnormal Child Psychology, 25,* 399–412.

Clarke-Stewart, K. A., Allhusen, V. D., McDowell, D. J., Thelen, L., & Call, J. D. (2003). Identifying psychological problems in young children: How do mothers compare with child psychiatrists? *Applied Developmental Psychology, 23,* 589–624.

Dowdy, E., & Kim, E. (2012). Choosing informants when conducting a universal screening for behavioral and emotional risk. *School Psychology Forum, 6*(4), 1–10.

Frick, P. J., Burns, C., & Kamphaus, R. W. (2009). *Clinical assessment of child and adolescent personality and behavior* (2nd ed.). New York: Springer

Goodman, R., Ford, T., Simmons, H., Gatward, R., & Meltzer, H. (2003). Using the strengths and difficulties questionnaire (SDQ) to screen for child psychiatric disorders in a community sample. *International Review of Psychiatry, 15,* 166–172.

Goodman, R., Ford, T., Corbin, T., & Meltzer, H. (2004). Using the strengths and difficulties questionnaire (SDQ) multi-informant algorithm to screen looked-after children for psychiatric disorders. *European Child and Adolescent Psychiatry, 13,* 11/25–11/31.

Goyette, C. H., Conners, C. K., & Ulrich, R. F. (1978). Normative data on revised conners parent and teacher rating scales. *Journal of Abnormal Child Psychology, 6,* 221–236.

Grietens, H., Onghena, P., Prinzie, P., Gadeyne, E., Van Assche, V., Ghesquiere, P., & Hellinckx, W. (2004). Comparison of mothers', fathers', and teachers' reports on problems behavior in 5- to 6-year-old children. *Journal of Psychopathology and Behavioral Assessment, 26,* 137–146.

Grills, A. E., & Ollendick, T. H. (2003). Multiple informant agreement and the anxiety disorders interview schedule for parents and children. *Journal of the American Academy of Child and Adolescent Psychiatry, 42,* 30–40.

Handwerk, M. L., Larzelere, R. E., Soper, S. H., & Friman, P. C. (1999). Parent and child discrepancies in reporting severity of problem behaviors in three out-of-home settings. *Psychological Assessment, 11,* 14–22.

Hill, L. G., Lochman, J. E., Coie, J. D., Greenberg, M. T., & The Conduct Problems Prevention Research Group. (2004). Effectiveness of early screening for externalizing problems: Issues of screening accuracy and utility. *Journal of Consulting and Clinical Psychology, 72,* 809–820.

Jensen, P. S., Rubio-Stipec, M., Canino, G., Bird, H. R., Dulcan, M. K., Schwab-Stone, M. E., & Lahey, B. B. (1999). Parent and child contributions to diagnosis of mental disorder: Are both informants always necessary? *Journal of the American Academy of Child and Adolescent Psychiatry, 38,* 1569–1579.

Johnston, C., & Murray, C. (2003). Incremental validity in the psychological assessment of children and adolescents, *Psychological Assessment, 15,* 496–507.

Jones, D., Dodge, K. A., Foster, E. M., Nix, R., & The Conduct Problems Prevention Research Group. (2002). Early identification of children at risk for costly mental health service use. *Prevention Science, 3,* 247–256.

Juechter, J. I., Dever, B. V., & Kamphaus, R. W. (2012). Mental health and academic outcomes in elementary school. *School Psychology Forum, 6,* 137–147.

Kamphaus, R. W., & Frick, P. J. (2002). *Clinical assessment of child and adolescent personality and behavior* (2nd ed.). Boston: Allyn & Bacon.

Kamphaus, R. W., & Reynolds, C. R. (2007). *Behavior assessment system for children-Second Edition (BASC-2): Behavioral and Emotional Screening System (BESS).* Bloomington: Pearson.

Kaufman, J., Cook, A., Arny, L., Jones, B., & Pittinsky, T. (1994). Problems defining resiliency: Illustrations from the study of maltreated children. *Development and Psychopathology, 6,* 215–229.

Kolko, D. J., & Kazdin, A. E. (1993). Emotional/behavioral problems in clinic and nonclinic children: Correspondence among children, parent, and teacher reports. *Journal of Child Psychology and Psychiatry, 34,* 991–1006.

Levitt, J. M., Saka, N., Romanelli, L. H., & Hoagwood, K. (2007). Early identification of mental health problems in schools: The status of instrumentation. *Journal of School Psychology, 45,* 163–191.

Lochman, J. E., & The Conduct Problems Prevention Research Group. (1995). Screening of child behavior problems for prevention programs at school entry. *Journal of Consulting and Clinical Psychology, 63,* 549–559.

Loeber, R., Green, S. M., & Lahey, B. B. (1990). Mental health professionals' perceptions of the utility of children, mothers, and teachers as informants on childhood psychopathology. *Journal of Clinical Child Psychology, 19,* 136–143.

Loeber, R., Green, S. M., Lahey, B. B., & Stouthamer-Loeber, M. (1991). Differences and similarities between children, mothers, and teachers as informants on disruptive child behavior. *Journal of Abnormal Child Psychology, 19,* 75–95.

McFall, R. M. (2005). Theory and utility—Key themes in evidence-based assessment: Comment on the special section. *Psychological Assessment, 17,* 312–323.

Mesman, J., & Koot, H. M. (2000). Child-reported depression and anxiety in preadolescence: I. Associations with parent- and teacher-reported problems. *Journal of the American Academy of Child and Adolescent Psychiatry, 39,* 1371–1378.

Pagano, M. E., Cassidy, L. J., Little, M., Murphy, J. M., & Jellinek, M. S. (2000). Identifying psychosocial dysfunction in school aged children: The Pediatric Symptom Checklist as a self-report measure. *Psychology in the Schools, 37,* 91–106.

Phillips, V., Nelson, C. M., & McLaughlin, J. R. (1993). Systems change and services for students with emotional/behavioral disabilities in Kentucky. *Journal of Emotional and Behavioral Disorders, 1,* 155–164.

Power, T. J., Andrews, T. J., Eiraldi, R. B., Doherty, B. J., Ikeda, M. J., DuPaul, G. J, & Landau, S. (1998). Evaluating attention deficit hyperactivity disorder using multiple informants: The incremental utility of combining teacher with parent reports. *Psychological Assessment, 10,* 250–260.

Reich, W., & Welner, Z. (1990). *The diagnostic interview for children and adolescents—revised (DICA–R).* Structured psychiatric interview. St. Louis: Washington University.

Renk, K. (2005). Cross-informant ratings of the behavior of children and adolescents: The "Gold Standard." *Journal of Child and Family Studies, 14,* 457–468.

Reynolds, C. R., & Kamphaus, R. W. (1992). *Behavior Assessment System for Children (BASC).* Circle Pines: Pearson.

Reynolds, C. R., & Kamphaus, R. W. (2004). *Behavior Assessment System for Children-second edition (BASC-2).* Circle Pines: Pearson.

Schanding, G. T. Jr, & Nowell, K. P. (2013). Universal screening for emotional and behavioral problems: Fitting a population-based model. *Journal of Applied School Psychology, 29*(1), 104–119.

Severson, H. H., Walker, H. M., Hope-Doolittle, J., Kratochwill, T. R., & Gresham, F. M. (2007). Proactive, early screening to detect behaviorally at-risk students: Issues, approaches, emerging innovations, and professional practices. *Journal of School Psychology, 45,* 193–223.

Simonian, S. J., & Tarnowski, K. J. (2001). Utility of the pediatric symptom checklist for behavioral screening of disadvantaged children. *Child Psychiatry and Human Development, 31,* 269–278.

Smith, S. R. (2007). Making sense of multiple informants in child and adolescent psychopathology: A guide for clinicians. *Journal of Psychoeducational Assessment, 25,* 139–149.

Sourander, A., Helstela, L., & Helenius, H. (1999). Parent-adolescent agreement on emotional and behavioral problems. *Social Psychiatry & Psychiatric Epidemiology, 34,* 657–663.

van der Ende, J. (1999). Multiple informants: Multiple views. In H. M. Koot, A. A. M. Crijnen, & R. F. Ferdinand (Eds.), *Child psychiatric epidemiology. Accomplishments and future directions* (pp. 39–52). Assen: Van Gorcum.

VanDeventer, M. C. (2008). *Universal emotional and behavioral screening for children and adolescents.* Unpublished doctoral dissertation.

Verhulst, F. C., Dekker, M. C., & van der Ende, J. (1997). Parent, teacher, and self-reports as predictors of signs of disturbance in adolescents: Whose information carries the most weight? *Acta Psychiatrica Scandinavica, 96,* 75–81.

Walker, H. M., & Severson, H. H. (1992). *Systematic Screening for Behavior Disorders (SSBD).* Longmont: Sopris West.

Walker, H., & Severson, H. (1994). Replication of the systematic screening for behavior disorders (SSBD) procedure for the identification of at-risk children. *Journal of Emotional and Behavioral Disorders, 2,* 66–78.

Walker, H. M., Severson, H., Stiller, B., Williams, G., Haring, N., Shinn, M., & Todis, B. (1988). Systematic screening of pupils in the elementary age range at risk for behavior disorders development and trial testing of a multiple gating model. *Remedial and Special Education, 9*(3), 8–20.

Walker, H. M., Small, J. W., Severson, H. H., Seeley, J. R., & Feil, E. G. (2014). Multiple-gating approaches in universal screening within school and community settings. In R. J. Kettler, T. A. Glover, C. A. Albers, & K. A. Feeney-Kettler (Eds.), *Universal screening in educational settings: Evidence-based decision making for schools* (pp. 47–75). Washington, DC: American Psychological Association.

Weisz, J. R., Sandler, I. N., Durlak, J. A., & Anton, B. S. (2005). Promoting and protecting youth mental health through evidence-based prevention and treatment. *American Psychologist, 60,* 628–648.

Werthamer-Larsson, L., Kellam, S. G., & Wheeler, L. (1991). Effect of first-grade classroom environment on shy behavior, aggressive behavior, and concentration problems. *American Journal of Community Psychology, 19,* 585–602.

Wolraich, M. L., Lambert, E. W., Bickman, L., Simmons, T., Doffing, M. A., & Worley, K. A. (2004). Assessing the impact of parent and teacher agreement on diagnosing attention-deficit hyperactivity disorder. *Developmental and Beahvioral Pediatrics, 25,* 41–47.

Youngstrom, E., Loeber, R., & Stouthamer-Loeber, M. (2000). Patterns and correlates of agreement between parent, teacher, and male adolescent ratings of externalizing and internalizing problems. *Journal of Consulting and Clinical Psychology, 68,* 1038–1050.

Chapter 7
An Example Using the BASC-2 Behavioral and Emotional Screening System (BESS)

In this chapter, we provide an example of a multiple-gated screening program that we have implemented in several school districts in the USA. First, we provide an overview of the assessments used from the *Behavior Assessment System for Children, Second Edition* (BASC-2; Reynolds and Kamphaus 2004) and how they have been designed in a way that lends itself to multiple gating. Second, we focus more specifically on the *BASC-2 Behavioral and Emotional Screening System* (BESS; Kamphaus and Reynolds 2007), as this is the screening instrument associated with the BASC-2 system and requires more careful attention, given the focus of this volume. Finally, we provide an overview of the implementation in the school districts, including lessons learned and examples of data reports.

The BASC-2 System of Assessment

The use of the BASC-2 omnibus assessment of behavioral and emotional difficulties as a diagnostic measure is widespread across school districts in the USA and is, therefore, an intuitive choice for integrating emotional and behavioral screening into existing school psychological services in many districts. The BASC-2 family of instruments (Reynolds and Kamphaus 2004) is composed of the self-report of personality (SRP), Parent Rating Scales (PRS), and Teacher Rating Scales (TRS), which assess the age range of 2½ through 18 years. The BASC-2 forms contain four subscales: externalizing problems, internalizing problems, school problems, and adaptive skills. A Behavioral Symptoms Index (BSI) is also provided and indicates overall behavioral and emotional problems across all measured domains. The BASC-2 TRS and PRS items are rated on a four-point frequency response scale, ranging from "Never" to "Almost Always." Both forms can be completed in approximately 20 minutes. The SRP, designed for ages 8 through 18 years, can be completed in 30–40 minutes. The SRP not only includes the same frequency response but also contains items that require a dichotomous "True" or "False" response. All BASC-2 forms were developed jointly in Spanish and English. Thus,

M. C. Stiffler, B. V. Dever, *Mental Health Screening at School*, Contemporary Issues in Psychological Assessment, DOI 10.1007/978-3-319-19171-3_7

the Spanish version is not a mere translation of the English form; its development is described in detail in the BASC-2 manual.

The BASC-2 norms were based on a large normative sample that is representative of the general population of US children with regard to sex, race/ethnicity, and clinical or special education classification (Reynolds and Kamphaus 2004). The BASC-2 manual provides three types of reliability evidence for the three informant choices: internal consistency, test–retest reliability, and inter-rater reliability. The manual presents evidence of factor analytic support for the construct validity of the scales and subscales. The BASC-2 instrument and its component scales also exhibit high correlations with analogous scales from other behavior rating scales (Reynolds and Kamphaus 2004, 1992). Additionally, several independent reviews of the BASC have noted that the BASC TRS and PRS possess adequate to good evidence of reliability and validity using a variety of indicators (Doyle et al. 1997; Vaughn et al. 1997).

One advantage of the BASC-2 is that it can be scored on the computer using the ASSIST Plus scoring software; computer hand-entry or scanned-entry are both available options. This software provides information regarding Diagnostic and statistical Manual-IV-Text Revision (DSM-IV-TR) (APA 2000) diagnostic criteria, which is a useful feature for those interested in diagnostic assessment. In addition, the ASSIST Plus software is integrated with the *BASC-2 Intervention Guide* (Vannest et al. 2008), generating data-based intervention guide narratives based on scale scores. This narrative provides a summary of up to two interventions for each identified problem area, including a classification of BASC-2 subscale scores into primary (i.e., *T*-score 70 or higher) and secondary intervention areas (i.e., *T*-score of 60–69). For each intervention, a brief summary is provided along with an example. Procedural steps for implementing the intervention are generated along with considerations for implementing the intervention and a list of research studies that report on the effectiveness of the intervention technique. A maximum of two evidence-based interventions for a total of three BASC-2 problem areas are printed in the intervention report.

The *Behavior Assessment System for Children-2 Intervention Guide (BASC-2 IG)* is a comprehensive compendium of research-based interventions that are appropriately matched to the specific problem area a child is experiencing. For each BASC-2 problem area, a comprehensive literature review was conducted using electronic databases in psychology and education. The research studies summarized in the "Evidence for Use" sections of the IG provide general support for the use of these intervention methodologies and promising validity evidence for the procedural steps included in the IG. Parent Tip Sheets (one for each problem area) were developed to further the involvement of parents in the intervention process. The tip sheets provide information about particular areas of elevated scores, as well as the strategies that may be implemented at home. The documentation checklist facilitates the recording of the steps that have been taken to remediate or manage a child's behavioral or emotional problems. In addition to recording the steps that have been taken with the child, it also includes a section that allows the teacher to record the fidelity of the intervention approaches that have been used. The Classroom Intervention Guide contains interventions for a variety of behavioral and emotional

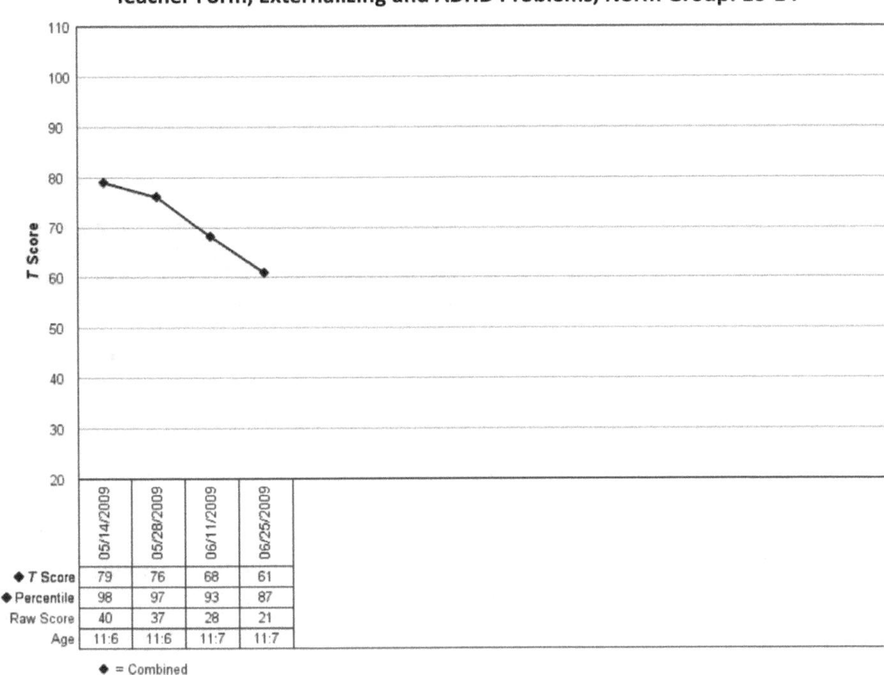

Fig. 7.1 Graph of BASC-2 PM data across four time-points

problems that can be used in a regular classroom setting. The classroom guide consists of two workbooks for two general types of behavioral or emotional problems: externalizing and school problems, and internalizing and adaptive skill problems.

Once intervention begins, progress can be monitored and recorded using the *BASC-2 Progress Monitor (BASC-2 PM*; Reynolds and Kamphaus 2009) form. Progress monitoring forms are available for teachers, parents, and students across four domains of interest: externalizing and attention deficit hyperactivity disorder (ADHD) problems, internalizing problems, social withdrawal, and adaptive skills. Each form contains 15–20 items, requiring not more than 5 minutes to complete and no informant training. As stated in Chapter 5, many times instruments that were designed for other purposes are used erroneously to monitor progress during intervention. However, the *BASC-2 PM* forms were designed to have the sensitivity necessary to detect the changes in each domain of interest specifically for the purpose of progress monitoring. Each form was developed using a nationally representative sample and has Spanish language versions available as well. Psychometric properties including internal consistency, test–retest reliability, and correlations with similar measures are adequate; full information is provided in the *BASC-2 PM* manual. The *BASC-2 PM* forms are scored using the *BASC-2 PM* ASSIST Plus software, which provides information about score elevation as compared to national norms, as well as the statistical significance of change in scores over time. Examples of the graphical and tabular information generated using the *BASC-2 PM* form over time are provided in Figs. 7.1 and 7.2. As shown in Fig. 7.1, this case demonstrated

Teacher Form, Externalizing and ADHD Problems, Norm Group: Ages 10-14

						Comparison to Baseline			Comparison to Previous Tests		
Test Date	Age	Raw Score	T Score	Percentile Rank	90% CI	Tests	Difference	Sig Level	Tests	Difference	Sig Level
T1: 05/14/2009	11:6	40	79	98	76-82	---	---	---	---	---	---
T2: 05/28/2009	11:6	37	76	97	73-79	T2-T1	-3	NS	---	---	---
T3: 06/11/2009	11:7	28	68	93	65-71	T3-T1	-11	.05	T3-T2	-8	.05
T4: 06/25/2009	11:7	21	61	87	58-64	T4-T1	-18	.05	T4-T3	-7	.05

Fig. 7.2 Example of BASC-2 PM data across four time-points

decreases in teacher-reported externalizing and ADHD problems over the course of approximately 6 weeks. Figure 7.2 provides information regarding the statistical significance of these changes and indicates that there was a significant difference between the behavioral ratings provided at Time 1 and Time 3. Clearly, this is a strong tool for use in monitoring progress, providing information regarding not only change but also the magnitude of any observed changes over time.

When used in concert with the *BASC-2 Behavioral and Emotional Screening System* (BESS; Kamphaus and Reynolds 2007), described in more detail in the next section, it is clear that the BASC-2 family of assessments was designed with a multiple-gated approach in mind. At the first gate, screening using the administration of the BESS to one or more informants establishes the pool of children and adolescents who are at elevated levels of risk for behavioral and emotional problems. At the second gate, those who were identified as at-risk on the BESS are rated by one or more informants on the complete BASC-2 in order to detect specific areas of difficulty as well as consider potential diagnostic classification; the reader is directed to Chapter 6 for more specific information regarding empirical support for this two-gated approach. Furthermore, the *BASC-2 Intervention Guide* provides suggested interventions that can be used both within the classroom and in a more individualized format. Completion of the *BASC-2 PM,* both before and during the intervention phase, assists with establishing a baseline in the domain of interest as well as monitoring the extent of progress over time. This complete recommended system of approach is represented in Fig. 7.3 with red arrows signifying continued risk/difficulty and green arrows representing students who exit the system at a given gate.

The BASC-2 Behavioral and Emotional Screening System

The *BASC-2 Behavioral and Emotional Screening System* (BESS) is a brief screening measure used to identify behavioral and emotional strengths and weaknesses in youth from preschool-age through high school (Kamphaus and Reynolds 2007) with the self-report appropriate for students in grades 3–12. Like the BASC-2, the

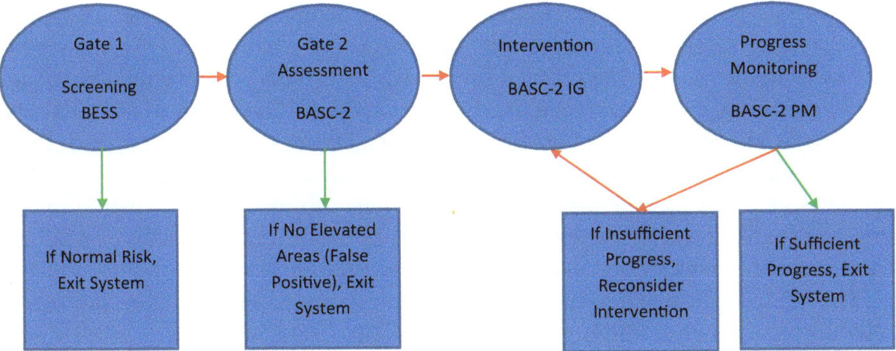

Fig. 7.3 Multiple-gated approach to using the BASC-2 system

BESS consists of three informant report forms (parent, teacher, and child/adolescent) and is available in English and Spanish versions. The BESS test development program was consistent with the definition of behavioral and emotional risk offered by the report of the National Academies (O'Connell et al. 2009): "For prevention, one of the goals of screening should be to identify communities, groups, or individuals exposed to risks or experiencing early symptoms that increase the potential that they will have negative emotional or behavioral outcomes and take action prior to there being a diagnosable disorder" (p. 223). Accordingly, for the purposes of BESS development, behavioral and emotional risk was defined as early symptoms that may later develop into disorders that reach diagnostic thresholds for special education placement or a mental health disorder. Therefore, it is important to note that the BESS was truly designed to be used as a brief, quick screening instrument for elevated risk and not as a comprehensive or diagnostic assessment tool.

Test developers designed the content of the items on the BESS to represent the major constructs of child adjustment (Reynolds and Kamphaus 2004; Kamphaus and Reynolds 2007): internalizing problems, externalizing problems, school problems, and adaptive skills. Items were selected by conducting a factor analysis on all items from the standardized pool of the BASC-2; items with the highest factor loadings were selected within each dimension on each form with roughly equal representation of the dimensions of the BASC-2 on each BESS screener. Additionally, in order to increase internal consistency within the internalizing factor the test developers chose several additional internalizing items to include on the BESS form based upon content validity.

The BESS teacher screener consists of 27 items, and the student and parent screeners consist of 30 items each. The BESS requires no informant training and can be completed in 5 minutes or less for each child to be rated. Respondents are given four rating options—Never, Sometimes, Often, or Almost Always—for each item and the sum of the items generates a total *T*-score with high scores reflecting greater problems (Kamphaus and Reynolds 2007). The scoring rubric or risk level for behavioral and emotional risk is as follows: (a) a *T*-score of 20–60 suggests a "normal" level of risk; (b) 61–70 suggests an "elevated" level of risk; and (c) 71 or higher suggests an "extremely elevated" level of risk. The risk level classification cut-scores were developed to maximize sensitivity and specificity, and results presented in the manual suggest that sensitivity, specificity, positive predictive value, and negative predictive value were generally high. The BESS may be entered by hand or via scanner with computer software. The software report includes raw scores, *T*-scores, and percentiles based on a normative sample that closely matches recent US Census population characteristics. This information is available for individual students and aggregated groups, such as classrooms, schools, or districts, for those who are interested in comparing screening results across multiple levels.

The BESS split-half reliability estimates range from 0.90 to 0.97. Test–retest reliability estimates are high, ranging from 0.80 to 0.91. Inter-rater reliability estimates range from 0.71 to 0.83. The concurrent validity of the BESS was examined by administering the items along with other social-emotional measures. In addition, the BESS provides validity indices to detect biased responding; the availability of these validity scales has been cited as a particular advantage of the BESS screener (Levitt et al. 2007).

Since its publication, other independent studies have also examined the factor structure and other psychometric properties of the BESS. Dowdy et al. (2011b) found that the Parent BESS loaded onto four distinct factors: externalizing problems, attention problems, internalizing problems, and adaptive skills. It is interesting to note that, in this instance, externalizing and attention problems separated from one another despite the fact that they were conceptualized as belonging to the same factor. Dowdy et al. (2011a) determined that the Student BESS also contained four factors. These factors were inattention/hyperactivity, internalizing problems, school problems, and personal adjustment and reflected the anticipated content of the self-report form. Finally, Dever et al. (2012) discovered the four latent factors that were anticipated within the BESS teacher-report form: externalizing problems, internalizing problems, school problems, and adaptive skills.

It has been demonstrated that the BESS student form has moderate to high levels of stability across a 4-year period (Dowdy et al. 2014) and exhibits measurement invariance across African American, Hispanic, and Caucasian (non-Hispanic) students (Raines 2011). Studies of the BESS teacher form have found that it exhibits measurement invariance when rating English language learners (Dowdy et al. 2011c), is a better tool than teacher nomination when used to identify students with behavioral and emotional risk (Dowdy et al. 2013a), and identifies proportions of students as expected given a population-based model of mental health concerns (Schanding and Nowell 2013). Finally, the BESS parent-report has shown moderate correlations with DSM diagnostic criteria suggesting that risk is indeed related to, but not necessarily indicative of, diagnostic categories (Dowdy et al. 2013b).

As empirical evidence on the BESS screener continues to be collected, school districts across the nation are beginning to utilize this instrument to identify students who may be at-risk for behavioral and emotional difficulties. In order to better understand the feasibility, technical adequacy, and implementation of a screening program such as this, the remainder of the chapter provides real-world examples of two different school districts utilizing the BESS, both alone and as part of a multiple-gated approach.

Examples of Screening Programs Using the BESS Form

In this section, we recount our experiences with two different school districts: (1) South District and (2) West District. It is important to note that both districts initiated the interest in a screening or multiple-gated program and approached us for technical assistance in their endeavors; as mental health screening is still a nascent field, such supports are often necessary to get a universal screening program "off the ground" for the first time. Below we provide insight into decisions that must be made, challenges that a district may face when implementing such an approach, and examples of ways in which the data can be used to aid schools and districts in correctly identifying students in need of additional support and interventions.

The Example of South District

South District is a predominantly African American district located in a small city in the Southeastern USA. The administrators in South District were keenly interested in the ability of a screening program to identify potential behavioral and emotional risk prior to the development of more severe concerns due to an increase in behavioral incidents within their high schools. Therefore, in this instance, the administrators chose to begin by screening all students (Gate 1) in four target high schools identified as having the highest number of disciplinary incidents. Approximately 3000 high school students were enrolled in the four high schools selected for participation in year 1.

The district wanted their results as quickly as possible in order to act on them immediately, and, therefore, chose to partner with our research program due to access to a scanning system for data entry. In a universal screening program, scannable data entry is almost a necessity as it decreases data entry and analysis time exponentially when compared to hand entry of hundreds or thousands of screening instruments. When considering what form of the BESS to administer, teachers expressed concerns about not knowing the students adequately because students changed classrooms throughout the day, and administrators expressed concerns about response rates if parents were selected to be the informants. Therefore, in order to maximize response rates and efficiency of data collection, the decision was made to use the self-report BESS form for all students. This is an instance where the practical concerns and constraints of the district were necessary to consider when determining the approach to screening that would be most acceptable to the district and its stakeholders.

As stated by Parisi et al. (2014), generating "buy in" is critical before beginning a screening program; this is especially true in the case of school psychologists, who in most cases will be responsible for interpreting the results of the assessment and making recommendations regarding next steps. Therefore, prior to the screening day, researchers and administrators met with school psychologists and interested teachers to explain the procedure and anticipated data that would be available following the screening. In this meeting, a plan was developed to screen all students in each school during their supervisory period in order to avoid loss of instructional time. In addition, the team decided to use individuals other than teachers to administer the screener in a group format so that students could be assured of the confidentiality of their individual responses. The district already had a passive consent procedure in place for any school-wide assessments, which included academic, behavioral, or health assessments. Although this district had a mechanism in place for passive consent, in other districts consent may be a roadblock to collecting universal data; this issue is discussed more fully in Chapter 8.

It should be noted that the preparation for screening is at least as important as, and perhaps more time-intensive than, the actual administration of the screening instruments. Prior to the screening day, teams prepared packets for each homeroom, including the appropriate number of instruments, pencils, and student rosters. A script was developed in order to ensure that all administrations would be carried out consistently across assistants (Dever et al. 2013). In this case, student rosters were used to check the accuracy of demographic information provided by the students following the administration of the BESS form; later we discuss a lesson learned from this example that suggests having screening team members use student rosters to complete particular sets of information prior to the screening day.

On the day of screening, research assistants and school psychologists administered the BESS forms to students in their homerooms; this process required only approximately 30 minutes of time per school. Following screening, forms were scanned in order to minimize the amount of time between screening and follow-up with those who were identified as being at elevated levels of risk. Using this method, within approximately 2 weeks all data were collected, scanned, and disseminated back to the schools.

The BESS software provides results for each student screened, which can be organized in a roster by classroom, school, or district. The results are presented such that students with the highest levels of risk appear at the top of the list, to assist with triage efforts. In Figure 7.4, we present a truncated version of the data provided to South District. Note that these data include information on each of the four validity indices, raw scores, *T*-scores, and risk-level classification. Given this information, South District was able to coordinate a comprehensive assessment (Gate 2) for each of the students who reported elevated levels of risk and were not currently receiving any services.

Additionally, we provided each of the four high schools with an aggregated report of its results at the school-level, broken down by gender and grade level. This school-level report provided information on the total numbers of students classified as at elevated or extremely elevated risk by grade level and gender. In addition, based on previous factor analytic work that suggested that the self-report BESS contains items that cover the domains of internalizing problems, inattention, school problems, and adaptive skills (Dowdy et al. 2011a), the school-level reports also provided information concerning aggregate levels in each of these four areas for all the students in that school. Figure 7.5 presents the results of risk level by grade for one particular school and indicates that students in the higher grades (11–12)

	Validity Indices			Scores		
Test Date	F	CONS	PTRN	Raw	T	Classification
12/1/14	E	A	A	64	83	Extremely Elevated
12/1/14	A	A	A	51	73	Extremely Elevated
12/1/14	A	A	A	50	72	Extremely Elevated
12/1/14	A	A	A	42	66	Elevated
12/1/14	A	A	L	35	61	Elevated
12/1/14	A	A	A	32	58	Normal
12/1/14	A	A	A	29	56	Normal
12/1/14	A	A	A	28	55	Normal
12/1/14	A	A	A	15	45	Normal

Fig. 7.4 Example of triaged BESS results for students, with names removed

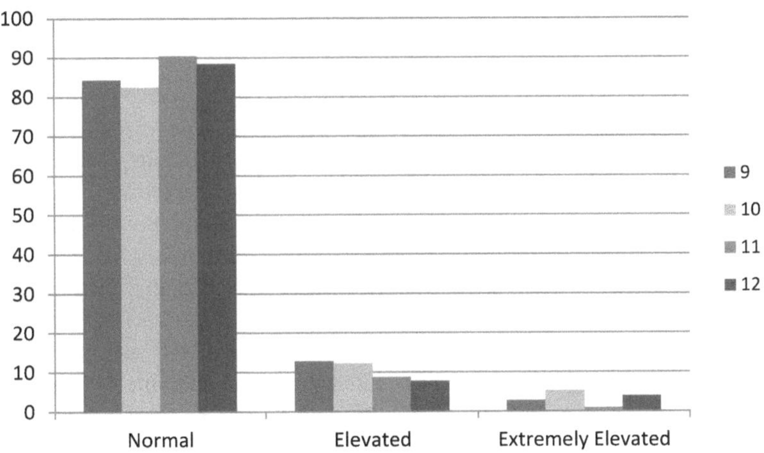

Fig. 7.5 Sample report of classification by grade

reported lower levels of risk. This finding resulted in school-wide discussions of ways to support the 9th and 10th grade students. This school was also informed that females reported higher levels of internalizing problems than males, but that there were no significant gender differences in the other domains (Fig. 7.6).

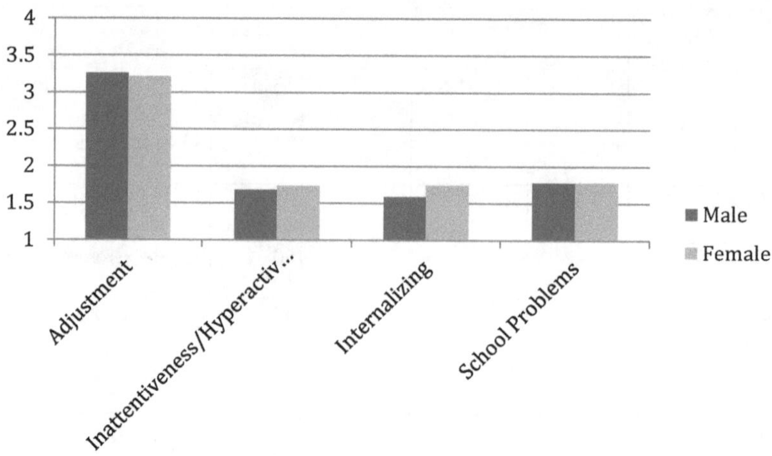

Fig. 7.6 Sample report of domain scores by gender

As Parisi et al. (2014) suggest, the practice of screening itself is often instrumental in gaining momentum for a screening program; without actually seeing the data about your own classrooms, schools, and districts, it is often difficult to visualize the impact that such data might have in a real-world application. After the presentation of results to the four selected high schools, the administrators, teachers, and school psychologists reported that they were able to see more clearly the utility of such data. Due to the overwhelming perception that the benefits of these screening data far outweighed the costs, South District decided to conduct universal screening at all of its high schools the following year. The process was the same as that described above with one exception: student rosters were used to complete student names and identification numbers on the BESS forms prior to the screening day. This decision was made after realizing that having the students complete this information themselves required more time than actually completing the BESS items themselves; therefore, screening time upon second implementation took approximately 15–20 minutes per administration rather than 30 minutes.

Figure 7.7 provides a poignant example of the type of data that district-level universal screening is able to provide. Across all high school students in South District, 10th grade students reported significantly higher levels of risk as compared to the other grades. As researchers, we had expected 9th grade students to have the highest levels of risk due to transitional difficulties. However, administrators at the high schools immediately understood this result given information that we as researchers did not have; namely, all high schools in the district provided smaller, school-within-a-school experiences for their 9th grade students in order to assist them in adjusting to the high school experiences. The screening data provided a different perspective according to these administrators: rather than aiding with adjustment, it seemed that students were experiencing delayed behavioral and emotional difficulties upon being integrated into the larger high school at grade 10. These data provided principals and assistant principals with the opportunity to rethink the current

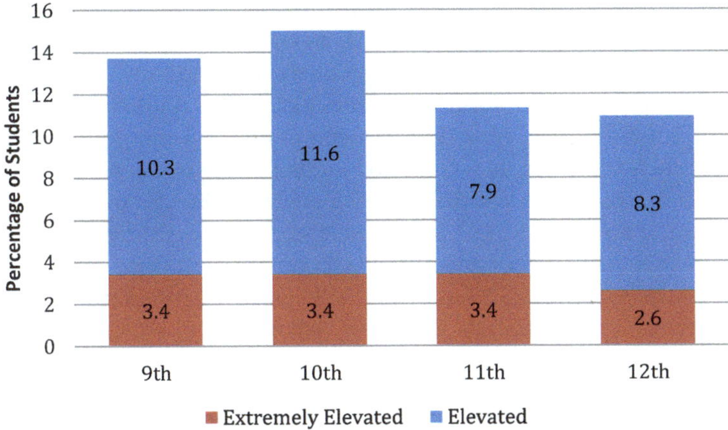

Fig. 7.7 District-level BESS results by grade

system by considering ways to integrate students into the high school incrementally throughout grades 9 and 10. As one principal so eloquently summarized regarding the BESS data, "With these data, I know how to meet the needs of my students… I feel like I am no longer committing random acts of leadership."

The Example of West District

West District is an urban, predominantly Latino, school district near the West Coast of the USA. This district was interested in universal screening in selected schools at the elementary, middle, and high school levels; therefore, different decisions were made regarding the procedures for screening given the need to screen across grades K-12. In elementary school, teacher- and parent-report forms were completed in year 1; however, in year 2, the parent-report forms were omitted at the elementary level due to a lower response rate than desired given the goal to screen universally. At the middle and high school levels, student-report forms were selected as the most appropriate and efficient consistent with the case of South District.

Like most large, urban districts across the country, teachers in this district were under tremendous pressure and had a long list of demands and responsibilities. As such, attempts were made to make the screening at the elementary level as palatable as possible (issues of social validity are discussed more extensively in Chapter 8). To demonstrate commitment to the screening effort, administrators at each selected elementary school dedicated one professional development meeting to the collection of BESS teacher-report data. Using this method, teachers did not have to bring any forms home to complete during their own time, and all the forms were finished in the same period allowing for efficiency in collection and entry of the data.

Preparation for screening, screening at the middle and high school levels, and data entry were conducted using the methodology described in the previous example. Based on what our team had learnt previously, student names and identification numbers were completed prior to the day of screening when possible in order to limit the amount of time needed for the screening procedure.

Although some BASC-2 forms were administered as follow-up assessments in the case of South District, West District more closely adhered to a multiple-gated system as described in Chapter 6. Following the administration of the BESS, all of the students who were identified as being at elevated levels of risk were further evaluated using a full BASC-2 assessment. Decisions regarding the choice of informant for this assessment were based both on research (e.g., teacher or parent among younger students and those with anticipated externalizing problems, student report among older students with likely internalizing problems) and practicality (e.g., whether the first chosen informant responded to the request to complete the BASC-2 form). Following the BASC-2 assessment, students who were already receiving appropriate services for their needs continued to be monitored. For those students who were not yet receiving services, appropriate interventions were implemented. In some instances, this included the development of new student groups focused on skill-building and self-monitoring. Currently, these groups are being conducted within the schools, and schools are collecting progress monitoring data on these groups using the BASC-2 PM measures most suitable given the goal of the group (e.g., students in a social skills group would likely complete a social withdrawal BASC-2 PM form). The efforts in West District present an applied example of school-wide implementation of the multiple-gated BASC-2 system as presented in Fig. 7.3. As we continue to collaborate with this district, we hope to learn more about the challenges and triumphs associated with this approach and its multiple components.

Conclusion

In this chapter, we provided an overview of the BASC-2 family of assessments within a multiple-gated screening framework. More specifically, we presented information on two applied examples with which we are familiar, given our provision of technical assistance to both the districts. Our use of the BASC-2 family of assessments was due both to our own expertise with these instruments as well as the desire of both the districts to continue with their use of these instruments; examples of research utilizing other screening measures and other multiple-gating systems are available in other chapters throughout this volume. Although more research is clearly needed about the BESS, BASC-2, and related instruments, the use of these assessments thus far provides promising results regarding their utility, acceptability, and feasibility, even among large, urban school districts.

References

American Psychiatric Association. (2000). *Diagnostic and statistical manual of mental disorders* (4th Ed., text rev.). Washington, DC: Author.

Dever, B. V., Mays, K. L., Kamphaus, R. W., & Dowdy, E. (2012). The factor structure of the BASC-2 behavioral and emotional screening system teacher form, child/adolescent. *Journal of Psychoeducational Assessment, 30*(5), 488–495.

Dever, B. V., Kamphaus, R. W., Dowdy, E., Raines, T. C., & DiStefano, C. (2013). Surveillance of middle and high school mental health risk by student self-report screener. *Western Journal of Emergency Medicine, 14*(4), 384.

Doyle, A., Ostrander, R., Skare, S., Crosby, R. D., & August, G. J. (1997). Convergent and criterion-related validity of the behavior assessment system for children-parent rating scale. *Journal of Clinical Child Psychology, 26*(3), 276–284.

Dowdy, E., Twyford, J. M., Chin, J. K., DiStefano, C. A., Kamphaus, R. W., & Mays, K. L. (2011a). Factor structure of the BASC–2 behavioral and emotional screening system student form. *Psychological Assessment, 23*(2), 379.

Dowdy, E., Chin, J. K., Twyford, J. M., & Dever, B. V. (2011b). A factor analytic investigation of the BASC-2 behavioral and emotional screening system parent form: Psychometric properties, practical implications, and future directions. *Journal of School Psychology, 49,* 265–280.

Dowdy, E., Dever, B. V., DiStefano, C., & Chin, J. (2011c). Screening for emotional and behavioral risk among students with limited English proficiency. *School Psychology Quarterly, 26,* 14–26.

Dowdy, E., Doane, K., Eklund, K., & Dever, B. V. (2013a). A comparison of teacher nomination and screening to identify behavioral and emotional risk. *Journal of Emotional and Behavioral Disorders, 21,* 127–137.

Dowdy, E., Kamphaus, R. W., Abdou, A. S., & Twyford, J. M. (2013b). Detection of symptoms of prevalent mental health disorders of childhood with the parent form of the behavioral and emotional screening system. *Assessment for Effective Intervention, 38*(3), 192–198.

Dowdy, E., Nylund-Gibson, K., Felix, E., Morovati, D., Carnazzo, K., & Dever, B. V. (2014). Long-term stability of screening for behavioral and emotional risk. *Educational and Psychological Measurement, 74*(3), 453–472.

Kamphaus, R. W., & Reynolds, C. R. (2007). *Behavior assessment system for children -Second Edition (BASC-2): Behavioral and emotional screening system (BESS)*. Bloomington: Pearson.

Levitt, J. M., Saka, N., Romanelli, L. H., & Hoagwood, K. (2007). Early identification of mental health problems in schools: The status of instrumentation. *Journal of School Psychology, 45,* 163–191.

O'Connell, M., Boat, T., & Warner, K. (2009). *Preventing mental, emotional, and behavioral disorders among young people: Progress and possibilities*. Washington, DC: National Academies Press.

Parisi, D. M., Ihlo, T., & Glover, T. A. (2014). Screening within a multitiered early prevention model: Using assessment to inform instruction and promote students' response to intervention. In R. J. Kettler, T. A. Glover, C. A. Albers, & K. A. Feeney-Kettler (Eds.), *Universal screening in educational settings: Evidence-based decision making for schools* (pp. 19–46). Washington, DC: American Psychological Association.

Raines, T. C. (2011). Screening as the great equalizer: Eliminating disproportionality in special education referrals. (Unpublished doctoral dissertation). Georgia State University, Atlanta, GA.

Reynolds, C. R., & Kamphaus, R. W. (1992). *Behavior Assessment System for Children* (BASC). Circle Pines: AGS.

Reynolds, C. R., & Kamphaus, R. W. (2004). *Behavior assessment system for children-Second Edition (BASC-2)*. Circle Pines: Pearson.

Reynolds, C. R., & Kamphaus, R. W. (2009). *BASC-2 Progress Monitor*. Minneapolis: NCS Pearson.

Schanding Jr, G. T., & Nowell, K. P. (2013). Universal screening for emotional and behavioral problems: Fitting a population-based model. *Journal of Applied School Psychology, 29*(1), 104–119.

Vannest, K. J., Reynolds, C., & Kamphaus, R. (2008). *BASC-2 Intervention Guide*. Minneapolis: Pearson.

Vaughn, M. L., Riccio, C. A., Hynd, G. W., & Hall, J. (1997). Diagnosing ADHD (predominantly inattentive and combine type subtypes): Discriminant validity of the behavior assessment system for children and the achenbach parent and teacher rating scales. *Journal of Clinical Child Psychology, 26(*4), 349–357.

Chapter 8
Current Issues and Future Directions in Mental Health Screening

Throughout this volume, we have presented current research and practice in mental health screening in schools as it presently stands. A corpus of prior work is beginning to form supporting the benefits of screening to early prevention and intervention work in schools; however, much remains unknown, even concerning many of the issues we have touched upon in this book. More research must be done in order to ensure that sound science guides the increasingly popular practice of screening children for behavioral and emotional problems in order to avoid untoward outcomes and maximize the benefits of the screening effort.

Assessing Criterion Validity of Screening Instruments

In Chapter 4, we introduced the reader to a multitude of specific and broadband behavior-rating scales and systems that have been used for mental health screening in schools. When using any screener, it is important that the screener is related to a particular outcome of interest; this is known as criterion validity. In reviewing the literature, researchers have utilized a number of outcome measures when assessing the criterion validity of different screeners. Although this research has yet to compare multiple screeners on the same criteria, initial measurement validation is also critical to current and future efforts in screening research. August et al. (1992) focused on functional impairment using measures of behavioral (using the Internalizing and Externalizing dimensions of the CBCL-PRF (Child Behavior Checklist-Parent Report Form; Achenbach 1991), social (using various subscales of the Walker-McConnell Scale of Social Competence and School Adjustment; Walker and McConnell 1995), and academic (using Woodcock-Johnson Tests of Achievement; McGrew and Woodcock 2001) adjustment. In this way, they could assess impairment independent of clinical diagnoses. An individual found to have functional

M. C. Stiffler, B. V. Dever, *Mental Health Screening at School*, Contemporary Issues in Psychological Assessment, DOI 10.1007/978-3-319-19171-3_8

impairments in any of these three areas would be positively identified when performing the ROC (Receiver Operating Characteristic) curve analysis.

Other possible criterion/outcome measures include other DSM-IV/DSM-V (Diagnostic and Statistical Manual of Mental Disorders-Fourth/Fifth Edition) (APA 1994, 2013) or ICD (International Classification of Diseases) (WHO 1993) diagnoses (Tarnopolsky et al. 1979; Winter et al. 1999), special education classifications, longer, validated parent and teacher behavior rating scales (Simonian and Tarnowski 2001), mental health referral and treatment histories (Saunders and Wojcik 2004), clinician or teacher-rated levels of impairment (Kelleher et al. 1999; Pagano et al. 2000; Saunders and Wojcik 2004), as well as diagnostic structured interviews such as the Structured Clinical Interview for DSM-IV (SCID-IV; Kobak et al. 1997; Leon et al. 1999; Pagano et al. 2000; Schmitz et al. 1999).

As McFall (2005, p. 318) explained "Only when both sides of the assessment equation have been nailed down is it possible to evaluate what, if anything, the total assessment effort has revealed. Unfortunately, criterion assessment has not received the attention to date that it requires." No "gold standard" presently exists in psychological assessment research (August et al. 1992; McFall 2005) and all commonly used criterion measures described previously have significant limitations.

For example, obtaining teacher's ratings of students as the criterion often leads one to suspect method variance since teachers are usually the respondent on the screening measure as well. Special education placement, another commonly used outcome measure, is of unknown reliability and validity and has been found to be determined by factors other than a child's academic performance or behavior in school, including a child's sex or race/ethnicity. Kim and Rowe (2004) found that children in special education and those in regular education had identical teacher ratings of their behavior, thus raising the question of why one child was "placed" and another was not (Kim and Rowe 2004). Lastly, the use of DSM diagnosis as an outcome measure is a common practice in psychological assessment literature; however, many of the diagnostic categories found in the DSM have yielded inter-diagnostician reliability estimates lower than the internal consistency estimate of most psychological assessment instruments (i.e., 97; Kamphaus and Frick 2002).

Due to the limitations of all outcomes measures, researchers must emphasize the need for replication when conducting this type of research. Researchers often recommend a "bootstrapping" approach, meaning that we must continually validate new measures against known inferior measures until enough evidence is accumulated to demonstrate that the new measure is superior. In this regard, Schmidt et al. (2004) have observed, "…philosophers of science have shown that it is possible to start with fallible indicators and gradually improve on them, simultaneously refining assessment of the construct (Meehl 1992, p. 141)." However, due to the practical limitations of most applications in schools, typically one measure has been used in isolation in each screening effort; therefore, little data exist comparing screening assessments on important criteria such as false positives, false negatives, and important outcomes following screening.

Assessing Consequential Validity

Ultimately, evidence of validity based on the consequences of screening will be necessary to defend its use. In order to be cost-effective (an issue described at greater length later in this chapter), early identification must lead to better behavioral and emotional outcomes for children than would be expected in the case of current typical service identification practices. Research must be done to assess whether the intended consequences of such a screening program come to fruition. In order to do this, it would be necessary to implement a school-wide or even district-wide screening program and evaluate the actual consequences longitudinally across a number of years. As described in Chapter 7, some districts are beginning to screen universally; our hope is that these districts continue this effort and allow their data to be used for research that could help to better inform future screening programs.

First, it would be important to determine that the screening instrument was being utilized as intended in order to avoid unintended consequences that could be associated with a positive screen. Due to the ease of administration, schools may be tempted to use the screener as a diagnostic tool rather than as an indication of possible risk. Screeners are inherently less broad-based, assessing a necessarily limited range of behaviors and emotions due to their shorter length. Moreover, in choosing cutoff scores for screeners, we allow more false positives since the screener is only supposed to be the first gate of a multiple-gate system of identification. Therefore, placing too much weight on a positive screen could be quite costly, both in terms of use of resources and mislabeling of children based on preliminary results.

Second, it is critical to make sure that certain children are not being identified more or less often than others as being at-risk for behavioral and emotional maladjustment. For example, if the screener is only identifying those children with externalizing problems and not those with internalizing problems such as anxiety or depression, then those children with internalizing problems would fail to receive the more comprehensive assessment and services that they potentially need. Past research has found that self-reports are especially useful in the identification of students who need intervention for less visible difficulties such as internalizing problems (Merrell et al. 2002). Future research should continue to examine the accuracy and rates of identification of children with various patterns of symptomology, particularly when the goal is broad-based screening for risk for a variety of behavioral or emotional difficulties.

It is also important to determine whether screening instruments overidentify children of specific demographics, including race and gender. In some instances, demographic characteristics have been found to predict special education placement better than academic performance or socioeconomic status (e.g., Hosp and Reschly 2004; Skiba et al. 2008). In terms of race, African American students are overrepresented in the Emotional Disturbance (ED) category of special education, most specifically, and in special education, more broadly (Ahram et al. 2011; Hosp and Reschly 2003; Jasper and Bouck 2013; MacMillan and Reschly 1998; Skiba et al. 2008). Males are also overrepresented in special education at a ratio of between 1.5:1 and 3.5:1 (Christenson et al. 1983; Coutinho and Oswald 2005), and are particularly at-risk for being referred to special education for behavioral problems (Bryan et al. 2012; Coutinho and Oswald 2005; Wallace et al. 2008). Therefore, if one of the goals of screening is to provide information prior to a special education referral, it is imperative that the screening instrument does not exacerbate, or even better, begins to ameliorate, current patterns of disproportionality associated with being referred to and ultimately receiving special education services for behavioral and emotional problems.

Lastly, we would want to evaluate how the children who are identified by the screening instrument as being at-risk are being served. What types of early interventions are in place in schools, and are these interventions addressing the needs that are being identified by the screening process and follow-up assessments? As Goodman et al. (2003) explained, "There would obviously be no point in identifying a greater proportion of children with psychiatric disorders in the community if the only consequence were greater access to ineffective treatments…even if treatments are effective, there is no point identifying more children in need of treatment if existing services are already overstretched and no resources are available" (p. 171).

In our own work in schools, linking screening results with appropriate interventions has admittedly been one of the most difficult challenges we have faced. In many instances, it is necessary to work within the intervention framework that already exists within the schools, as many districts lack the time and resources required to develop new interventions based on screening results. However, it is also true that very little research has been conducted regarding the best steps to take following a positive screening, including intervention decisions. As stated by Vannest (2012), following a screening effort the school must make decisions regarding whom to serve, when to serve them, what service to provide, and who will provide that service. Vannest et al. (2008) compiled a compendium of empirically-validated interventions for various behavioral and emotional challenges; however, teacher training is often necessary, many interventions may be useful for only one specific difficulty, and schools may find it difficult to address all of the needs of children simultaneously. More research is needed concerning matching interventions to specific difficulties, focusing on progress over time. In addition, research on the impact of group interventions or school-wide prevention efforts on student outcomes over time could be useful for providing schools with limited resources with more efficient alternatives to address the needs of the students. This type of longitudinal research is costly and time-intensive; however, it is a crucial step in evaluating the long-term effectiveness of a universal screening program.

Assessing the Usefulness of Multiple-Gated Systems and Available Informants

In Chapter 6, we discussed the available research concerning multiple-gated approaches to screening, as well as choosing an informant for the screening assessment. Presently, there is no consensus regarding either the best number of gates, or the procedures to be implemented at each gate. Although some systems use three gates (e.g., Systematic Screening for Behavior Disorders (SSBD); Walker and Severson 1992), others have suggested two gates are sufficient (e.g., VanDeventer 2008; see Chapter 6 for a full review of the literature on this issue). Longitudinal studies of multiple-gated screening procedures are particularly crucial for determining the false negative and false positive rates of each configuration of gates to identify children who later develop significant behavioral and emotional problems.

Similarly, the best use of various informants, whether in a multiple-gated system or individually, when screening is still undecided. As reviewed in Chapter 6, the choice of informant(s) may depend upon the behavior of interest, as well as the age of the child and other characteristics of the potential informant(s). For example, teachers and parents may be best suited to provide information about younger children, particularly regarding their externalizing behaviors (Loeber et al. 1990). However, older children and adolescents may be the best source of information concerning their own internalizing problems (Loeber et al. 1991; Pagano et al. 2000; Smith 2007; Youngstrom et al. 2000).

Realistically, decisions regarding the number of gates and choice of informants are often driven by feasibility within a given setting. For example, among children who are just beginning at a new school setting (e.g., kindergarten), asking parents to complete screening forms at a registration event could serve as an efficient method of gathering information universally. However, for students in the 11th grade, it might be more difficult to send forms home to parents and have them successfully completed and returned to the school; in that instance, teacher- or student-reports completed on-site often yield a higher response rate and therefore, decrease the likelihood of students who are in need of follow-up assessment from "falling through the cracks" at the screening stage. As described in Chapter 7, student-report screening among middle and high school students may be more acceptable to teachers, as students often have multiple teachers in these grades, which makes identifying the "best" teacher informant a practical challenge.

To be most successful, practice must inform future research as much as research must inform future practice regarding the feasibility of collecting information over multiple gates, and/or from multiple informants. Researchers must seek out school districts who are already using multiple- or single-gated approaches to screening to better understand the implementation challenges that schools face when undertaking a screening effort (e.g., Dever et al. 2012). Even the strongest of research findings is not useful if it has limited external validity or generalizability to a real-world situation of the actual practice of screening in schools; therefore, the development of future best practices should include strong partnerships between researchers and school districts. Only with such applied work can researchers begin to understand the feasibility and utility of multiple-gated systems and the number and types of informants that are both necessary and plausible to involve in the process.

Assessing the Stability of Screening Results over Time

When embarking upon a universal screening program, it is important to consider a long-term plan for integrating screening into the procedures of a school or district. One decision that is frequently overlooked is how often the school or district will screen. Screening data are excellent for providing a snapshot of risk for behavioral and emotional problems at one point of time. However, these sorts of issues are often fluid and may depend upon individual and contextual circumstances at any given time; as such, future research is necessary for determining the frequency with which screening should be conducted in order to maximize classification accuracy, minimize false negatives, and reduce costs (an issue to be discussed further in the next section).

Although previous research suggests that behavioral and emotional problems are fairly stable across time (Essex et al. 2009; Levitt et al. 2007), there is limited empirical knowledge regarding the stability of screening scores and classifications (at-risk vs. not at-risk) over time. Some scholars in the field have recommended that screening should occur three times per year in order to identify students who may need additional services, those whose functioning may have deteriorated over time, and new students who may be in need of support (Parisi et al. 2014; Walker et al. 2014). Walker (2010) suggested that screening for behavioral and emotional risk take place once early in the academic year, with a follow-up screening only for schools with higher student transiency in the early spring in order to avoid missing any new students who have transferred into the school and might be in need of services.

Dowdy and colleagues examined the stability of screening scores and found that behavioral and emotional risk screening classifications were moderately stable across a 4-year period (Dowdy et al. 2014b). Moderate stability coefficients were also found for both overall risk and for domains of risk (internalizing, externalizing, adaptive skills, and school problems) in a district-wide effort across 2 years (Dever et al. in press). These empirical studies call into question the need for multiple screenings within the same academic year. However, there is a continued need to examine screening frequency and the stability of screening scores to determine the optimal screening schedule for schools and districts with the simultaneous goals of maximizing efficiency and minimizing risk to students. As service delivery decisions are often made based on these results, the frequency of screening is an important issue to evaluate in future research.

Assessing the Cost/Benefit Ratio

When evaluating potential screening tools, the accuracy of identification is critical to gathering good data; however, in the context of actual schools, the practicality of the instrument is also of utmost importance. One must balance the amount of information needed to reliably identify those children who are at-risk for emotional and behavioral problems against the time and monetary resources of those schools and districts that will be collecting the information. The scientific literature indicates that the impracticality of many screening measures has largely contributed to their lack of adoption on a wide scale in both pediatric and school settings (Flanagan et al. 2003; Saunders and Wojcik 2004; Schmitz et al. 1999). Therefore, one must compare the time and cost of adding additional levels of assessment and informants against the benefits that are gained in terms of increased accuracy of identification with each additional cost. For example, when an informant or gate is eliminated in a screening design, the number of children receiving full diagnostic assessments and more intensive interventions at a later time will likely increase due to the decrease in early identification and prevention procedures.

Researchers must consider what school personnel will tolerate in terms of time and financial investment. Teachers, school psychologists, administrators, and other educational stakeholders are extremely busy and their time is valuable. If the screening process takes too long for teachers to complete, universal screening is unlikely to be adopted successfully. Moreover, the costs associated with implementing a universal emotional and behavioral screening program, including personnel and materials costs, should be thoroughly examined. A cost–benefit ratio between the resources needed to conduct the screening program and the amount of information needed to make accurate predictions is a necessary step to future research.

Before embarking upon a universal screening program, school psychologists and other school personnel commonly express concerns about the "cost" of identifying a large number of students who will be left unable to be served by them (Dever et al. 2012). This concern is understandable, given the plethora of duties with which schools are tasked on a daily basis. However, upon presenting the data back to schools and districts, it has been our experience that most students who are identified as at-risk are already receiving services; therefore, the best approach for these students may be to merely monitor their progress rather than a full reevaluation or change in intervention. According to a population-based model, we should expect approximately 20 % of students to be rated at elevated levels of risk; although somewhat anecdotal, we have found that only about 20 % of this 20 %, or about 4 % of total students screened, emerge as new cases that have not been previously identified or are not currently receiving services. For some of these students, a more comprehensive assessment might reveal that the screening result was a false positive; for others, this is a true positive result, and early intervention efforts should be considered before the detected risk worsens.

In general, research is need to determine whether a universal screening program adds to the burdens that teachers, school psychologists, and others already face or alleviates burdens of financial expense and time by increasing accuracy of referral and identifying children earlier. Presumably, accurate screening will decrease the need for time- and money-consuming procedures such as special education referral and full evaluations as well as more intensive interventions. However, empirical evidence is needed to support, or refute, this assumption concerning the relative costs and benefits of a universal screening program.

Addressing Perceptions of Screening

As demonstrated by several high profile legal actions and parental complaints regarding emotional and behavioral screening, public perceptions of screening must be addressed. One concern is that asking questions about suicidal intent may entice adolescents to actively consider suicide when they would have not done so otherwise. Gould et al. (2005) recently evaluated the iatrogenic risk of youth suicide screening programs and found no evidence to suggest that this is the case. In fact, their findings suggest that the screening may have been beneficial for students with symptoms of depression or previous suicide attempts. Although scientific research has not supported the hypothesis of iatrogenic risk of youth suicide screening programs, this public fear represents a significant barrier to public acceptance of universal emotional and behavioral screening of children and adolescents. In August 2003, Illinois was the first state to pass legislation in which a plan, drafted by the *Illinois Children's Mental Health Partnership* (ICMHP), recommended that "all children receive periodic social and emotional developmental screens" (Barlas 2004). This plan was met with great opposition by a group of parents who felt that, according to Barbara Shaw, chairman of the (ICMHP), "the schools have no place futzing with their children's mental health." The parents feared that emotional and behavioral screening would lead to the unnecessary labeling and medicating of their children. These occurrences suggest that public opinion of mental health disorders and our ability to detect and treat them may not yet be at the point where universal emotional and behavioral screening would be widely accepted.

Issues regarding the use of active or passive consent for collecting information on behavioral and emotional risk from students could have an influence on public perception and must be considered prior to the implementation of a universal screening program. Concerns regarding parental rights, student assent, and confidentially must be addressed explicitly prior to any screening effort. Active consent requires signed, explicit permission from a parent or guardian prior to screening his/her child; passive permission provides the parent or guardian with the opportunity to withdraw his/her child from the screening, with a nonresponse indicative of the passive provision of permission. In the US, it is common for school districts to screen for vision, hearing, and academic concerns routinely with only passive or implied consent procedures in place. However, as Gardner (2011) made clear, behavioral and emotional health screening information may be considered more sensitive than those other domains, both by parents and the local jurisdiction; therefore, in some circumstances, active consent may be necessary prior to beginning any screening. The impact of an active versus passive consent procedure on response rate, and by extension, hit rate of identification has not yet been examined empirically; future practice could benefit from such an examination of the strengths and limitations of each type of consenting process on a screening effort.

In addition to public perceptions of screening, it is important for future research to collect information about the perceptions of educational stakeholders concerning screening procedures. Social validity refers to teachers' and others' beliefs that the procedures being conducted are both feasible and useful. Some research has found that while teachers perceive screening as useful and acceptable overall, they have concerns regarding feasibility of both universal screening and intervention efforts following screening (Greer et al. 2012). Social validity is critical to the ultimate success of a screening program, as it has been related to fidelity of implementation of school-based programming (e.g., Lane et al. 2009). Therefore, it is imperative for researchers to consider ways to improve social validity of screening work in order for such research to be implemented well in practical settings.

Finally, the buy-in of school leadership is necessary prior to starting a screening program, as the results of screening must be integrated into the procedures of a school or district in order to have any sort of meaningful impact on the school level (Parisi et al. 2014). In the best-case scenario, screening data would be used in a comprehensive data-based decision-making model concerning prevention and intervention for behavioral and emotional problems at the school- and/or district-levels. For this to become a reality, school leaders must be dedicated to the universal screening effort as an iterative process rather than an isolated incident. Past work has found that consensus or near consensus (e.g., 80 % or higher) is not necessarily needed among school personnel prior to beginning the screening program, but that a well-executed screening effort with clear results and strong leadership behind it can actually increase buy-in for subsequent screening (Parisi et al. 2014). As school psychologists are often the best-prepared in the areas of assessment, interpretation, and intervention, the commitment of the school psychologist to the screening program is essential (Dever et al. 2012). Despite the knowledge of the importance of school administrators and school psychologists for the success of a universal screening program, there is limited research on *how* to increase the commitment of these stakeholders. In the future, it is imperative that these issues be studied empirically in order to identify areas that could be strengthened or emphasized when introducing a new district or new personnel to the potential of universal screening to improve their students' behavioral, emotional, and ultimately, academic, outcomes.

Considering the Diversity of the Student Population

The growing diversity of students enrolled in US schools and the globalization of education in general, requires a consideration of how to engage in screening, assessment, and intervention efforts with diverse children and families in a culturally competent manner. The behavioral and emotional constructs of interest when screening are often influenced by and defined differently within each culture (Yates et al. 2008). Therefore, cultural information must be integrated into the screening process in order to avoid labeling behaviors that are normative in one culture as maladaptive (Dowdy et al. 2014a). In addition, the language abilities of the student being assessed, as well as any family members as informants, must be considered when determining the best way to collect screening information. Dowdy et al. (2014a) have recommended that informants who are English language learners are screened in their native language and preferred modality (i.e., oral vs. written). In addition, the language and reading level of consent forms must be appropriate for the selected informants. When screening among linguistically diverse populations, it is essential that measures are not simply translated from the languages in which they were originally developed to the new language as this may have an unexpected effect on the psychometric properties, meaning, and interpretation of the measure. As such, when designing a screening program the school or district should choose instruments for which there is evidence of appropriateness and psychometric properties within the entire population that is going to be screened (Dowdy et al. 2014a).

When the decision is made to use screening measures with a different population from that on which the measures were originally normed, there must be evidence of measurement invariance for the newly-intended population. In other words, one must ask whether the assessment is still measuring the domains of interest, with the same precision and accuracy, when the assessment is applied to a new group of students. Measurement invariance is important both when translating instruments to a new language, and when using an instrument in the same language, but among a new group of students. For example, if a screening instrument was developed and normed among a sample of students who were in middle school and 95 % Caucasian American, a researcher must consider whether that instrument performs the same psychometrically in a high school whose student body is 80 % African American, prior to interpreting the results within this new context.

Measurement invariance is emerging as an important venue for continued research in screening. Some researchers have provided preliminary evidence of measurement invariance of omnibus rating scales (e.g., *Child Behavior Checklist (CBCL);* Gross et al. 2006) and screening instruments (e.g., *BASC-2 Behavioral and Emotional Screening System*; Dowdy et al. 2011; Raines 2011) across language translations, racial and ethnic groups, and gender. However, much more work is needed in this area. Since inferences are made based on the outcome of screening, it is imperative that the instrument of choice is not biased against, or toward, the identification of certain students based on linguistic and cultural characteristics. Otherwise, screening results may serve to perpetuate the disproportionate representation of students that is currently seen in our referral and service systems in schools.

In some instances, practitioners may develop locally-based norms to make screening decisions as opposed to national norms that may not adequately represent the diversity of their own student body (Dowdy et al. 2014a). Local norms have the benefit of identifying the students with the most need in comparison to one's own local population (Glover and Albers 2007). However, national norms have the benefit of comparing a student's results to similar peers in one's own grade level, age group, or gender group. Research is needed to compare and contrast the results of screening efforts utilizing local and national norms in order to understand the circumstances under which each method might be the most appropriate and useful.

Conclusions and Final Thoughts

In this volume, we have attempted to compile the existing evidence regarding best practice and recommendations for screening based on empirical research. Although the rich history of mental health screening is clear, the concept of screening universally for risk for behavioral and emotional disorders has just come to the forefront of school psychology research and practice in the past decade or so. In this nascent field, there is much opportunity for further research regarding screening instruments, multiple-gated systems, choice of informants, and other relevant issues related to creating a comprehensive screening-to-intervention system.

Although such a turn-key system is yet to be developed, the field of mental health screening in schools has grown exponentially in the past few years, and this growth is likely to continue. The goals of prevention and early intervention fit well within an RtI framework and make sense intuitively, given the desire to address and ultimately ameliorate behavioral and emotional problems among students as early as possible. Great strides have been made concerning the development of screening instruments, their application in real-world school settings, and their links to intervention efforts; despite this progress, the field of mental health screening in schools remains an area that is "ripe for the picking" among researchers in the area of school psychology. Our hope is that this book will inspire both practitioners and researchers to continue to work toward establishing universal screening for behavioral and emotional risk in schools as typical, rather than exceptional, practice.

References

Achenbach, T. M. (1991). *Integrative Guide to the 1991 CBCL/4-18, YSR, and TRF Profiles*. Burlington: University of Vermont, Department of Psychology.

Ahram, R., Fergus, E., & Noguera, P. (2011). Addressing racial/ethnic disproportionality in special education: Case studies of suburban school districts. *Teachers College Record, 113*(10), 2233–2266.

American Psychiatric Association. (1994). *Diagnostic and statistical manual of mental disorders* (4th ed.). Washington, DC: Author.

American Psychiatric Association. (2013). *Diagnostic and statistical manual of mental disorders* (5th ed.). Washington, DC: Author.

August, G. J., Ostrander, R., & Bloomquist, M. J. (1992). Attention deficit hyperactivity disorder: Epidemiological screening method. *American Journal of Orthopsychiatrics, 62,* 387–396.

Barlas, S. (2004). Illinois passes controversial child screening plan. *Psychiatric Times, 21.* http://www.psychiatrictimes.com/articles/illinois-passes-controversial-child-screening-plan. Accessed 26 June 2015.

Bryan, J., Day-Vines, N. L., Griffin, D., & Moore-Thomas, C. (2012). The disproportionality dilemma: Patterns of teacher referrals to school counselors for disruptive behavior. *Journal of Counseling and Development, 90*(2), 177–190.

Christenson, S., Ysseldyke, J. E., Wang, J. J., & Algozzine, B. (1983). Teachers' attributions for problems that result in referral for psychoeducational evaluation. *The Journal of Educational Research, 76,* 174–180.

Coutinho, M. J., & Oswald, D. P. (2005). State variation in gender disproportionality in special education findings and recommendations. *Remedial and Special Education, 26*(1), 7–15.

Dever, B. V., Raines, T. C., & Barclay, C. M. (2012). Chasing the unicorn: Practical implementation of universal screening for behavioral and emotional risk. *School Psychology Forum, 6*(4), 108–118.

Dever, B. V., Dowdy, E., Raines, T. C., & Carnazzo, K. (In Press). Stability and change of behavioral and emotional screening scores. *Psychology in the Schools.*

Dowdy, E., Dever, B. V., DiStefano, C., & Chin, J. (2011). Screening for emotional and behavioral risk among students with limited English proficiency. *School Psychology Quarterly, 26,* 14–26.

Dowdy, E., Kamphaus, R. W., Twyford, J., & Dever, B. V. (2014a). Culturally competent screening approaches and treatments. In M. Weist, N. Lever, C. Bradshaw, & J. Owens (Eds). *Handbook of School Mental Health* (2nd ed.). New York: Springer.

Dowdy, E., Nylund-Gibson, K., Felix, E., Morovati, D., Carnazzo, K., & Dever, B. V. (2014b). Long-term stability of screening for behavioral and emotional risk. *Educational and Psychological Measurement, 74*(3), 453–472. doi:10.1177/0013164413513460.

Essex, M. J., Kraemer, H. C., Slattery, M. J., Burk, L. R., Boyce, W. T., Woodward, H. R., & Kupfer, D. J. (2009). Screening for childhood mental health problems: Outcomes and early identification. *Journal of Child Psychology and Psychiatry, 50*(5), 562–570.

Flanagan, K. S., Bierman, K. L., & Kam, C. M. (2003). Identifying at-risk children at school entry: the usefulness of multibehavioral problem profiles. *Journal of Clinical Child and Adolescent Psychology, 32,* 396–407.

Gardner, N. (2011). Potentials and impediments to universal, school-based screening for behavioral and emotional risk: A critical discourse analysis of current case law. (Unpublished doctoral dissertation). Georgia State University, Atlanta, GA.

Glover, T. A., & Albers, C. A. (2007). Considerations for evaluating universal screening assessments. *Journal of School Psychology, 45*(2), 117–135.

Goodman, R., Ford, T., Simmons, H., Gatward, R., & Meltzer, H. (2003). Using the strengths and difficulties questionnaire (SDQ) to screen for child psychiatric disorders in a community sample. *International Review of Psychiatry, 15,* 166–172.

Gould, M. S., Marrocco, F. A., Kleinman, M., Thomas, J. G., Mostkoff, K., Cote, J., & Davies, M. (2005). Evaluating iatrogenic risk of youth suicide screening programs. *Journal of the American Medical Association, 293,* 1635–1643.

Greer, F. W., Wilson, B. S., DiStefano, C., & Liu, J. (2012). Considering social validity in the context of emotional and behavioral screening. *School Psychology Forum, 6*(4), 148–159.

Gross, D., Fogg, L., Young, M., Ridge, A., Cowell, J. M., Richardson, R., & Sivan, A. (2006). The equivalence of the Child Behavior Checklist/1 1/2–5 across parent race/ethnicity, income level, and language. *Psychological Assessment, 18*(3), 313–323.

Hosp, J. L., & Reschly, D. J. (2003). Referral rates for intervention or assessment a meta-analysis of racial differences. *The Journal of Special Education, 37*(2), 67–80.

Hosp, J. L., & Reschly, D. J. (2004). Disproportionate representation of minority students in special education: Academic, demographic, and economic predictors. *Exceptional Children, 70*(2), 185–199.

Jasper, A. D., & Bouck, E. C. (2013). Disproportionality among African American students at the secondary level: Examining the MID disability category. *Education and Training in Autism and Developmental Disabilities, 48*(1), 31–40.

Kamphaus, R. W., & Frick, P. J. (2002). *Clinical assessment of child and adolescent personality and behavior* (2nd ed.). Boston: Allyn & Bacon.

Kelleher, K. J., Moore, C. D., Childs, G. E., Angelilli, M. L., & Comer, D. M. (1999). Patient race and ethnicity in primary care management of child behavior problems. *Medical Care, 37,* 1092–1104.

Kim, S., & Rowe, E. (2004, April). Similar risks, dissimilar outcomes: Rethinking risk in educational context. Paper presented at the annual conference of the American Educational Research Association, San Diego, CA.

Kobak, K. A., Taylor, L. vH., Dottl, S. L., Greist, J. H., Jefferson, J. W., Burroughs, D., Katzelnick, D. J., & Mandell, M. (1997). Computerized screening for psychiatric disorders in an outpatient community mental health clinic. *Psychiatric Services, 48,* 1048–1057.

Lane, K. L., Kalberg, J. R., Bruhn, A. L., Driscoll, S. A., Wehby, J. H., & Elliott, S. N. (2009). Assessing social validity of school-wide positive behavior support plans: Evidence for the reliability and structure of the primary intervention rating scale. *School Psychology Reviewer, 38,* 135–144

Leon, A. C., Kathol, R., Portera, L., Farber, L., Olfson, M., Lowell, K. N., & Sheehan, D. V. (1999). Diagnostic errors of primary care screens for depression and panic disorder. *International Journal of Psychiatry in Medicine, 29,* 1–11.

Levitt, J. M., Saka, N., Romanelli, L. H., & Hoagwood, K. (2007). Early identification of mental health problems in schools: The status of instrumentation. *Journal of School Psychology, 45,* 163–191.

Loeber, R., Green, S. M., & Lahey, B. B. (1990). Mental health professionals' perceptions of the utility of children, mothers, and teachers as informants on childhood psychopathology. *Journal of Clinical Child Psychology, 19,* 136–143.

Loeber, R., Green, S. M., Lahey, B. B., Stouthamer-Loeber, M. (1991). Differences and similarities between children, mothers, and teachers as informants on disruptive child behavior. *Journal of Abnormal Child Psychology, 19,* 75–95.

MacMillan, D. L., & Reschly, D. J. (1998). Overrepresentation of minority students the case for greater specificity or reconsideration of the variables examined. *The Journal of Special Education, 32*(1), 15–24.

McFall, R. M. (2005). Theory and utility—key themes in evidence-based assessment: Comment on the special section. *Psychological Assessment, 17,* 312–323.

McGrew, K. S., & Woodcock, R. W. (2001). *Technical manual. Woodcock-Johnson III.* Itasca: Riverside Publishing.

Meehl, P. E. (1992). Factors and taxa, traits and types, differences of degree and differences in kind. *Journal of Personality, 60*(1), 117–174.

Meehl, P. E., & Rosen, A. (1955). Antecedent probability and the efficiency of psychometric signs, patterns, or cutting scores. *Psychological Bulletin, 52,* 194–216.

Merrell, K. W., McClun, L. A., Kempf, K. G., & Lund, J. (2002). Using self-report assessment to identify children with internalizing problems: Validity of the internalizing symptoms scale for children. *Journal of Psychoeducational Assessment, 20*(3), 223–239.

Pagano, M. E., Cassidy, L. J., Little, M., Murphy, J. M., & Jellinek, M. S. (2000). Identifying psychosocial dysfunction in school aged children: The Pediatric Symptom Checklist as a self-report measure. *Psychology in the Schools, 37,* 91–106.

Parisi, D. M., Ihlo, T., & Glover, T. A. (2014). Screening within a multitiered early prevention model: Using assessment to inform instruction and promote students' response to intervention. In R. J. Kettler, T. A. Glover, C. A. Albers, & K. A. Feeney-Kettler (Eds.), *Universal screening in educational settings: Evidence-based decision making for schools* (pp. 19–46). Washington, DC: American Psychological Association.

Raines, T. C. (2011). Screening as the great equalizer: Eliminating disproportionality in special education referrals. (Unpublished doctoral dissertation). Georgia State University, Atlanta, GA.

Saunders, S. M. & Wojcik, J. V. (2004). The reliability and validity of a brief self-report questionnaire to screen for mental health problems: the health dynamics inventory. *Journal of Clinical Psychology in Medical Settings, 11,* 233–241.

Schmidt, N. B., Kotov, R., & Joiner, T. E. (2004). *Taxometrics: Toward a new diagnostic scheme for psychopathology.* Washington, DC: American Psychological Association.

Schmitz, N., Kruse, J., Heckrath, C., Alberti, L., & Tress, W. (1999). Diagnosing mental disorders in primary care: the General Health Questionnaire (GHQ) and the Symptom Check List (SCL-90-R) as screening instruments. *Social Psychiatry and Psychiatric Epidemiology, 34,* 360–367.

Simonian, S. J., & Tarnowski, K. J. (2001). Utility of the pediatric symptom checklist for behavioral screening of disadvantaged children. *Child Psychiatry and Human Development, 31,* 269–278.

Skiba, R. J., Simmons, A. B., Ritter, S., Gibb, A. C., Rausch, M. K., Cuadrado, J., & Chung, C. (2008). Achieving equity in special education: History, status, and current challenges. *Exceptional Children, 74*(3), 264–288.

Smith, S. R. (2007). Making sense of multiple informants in child and adolescent psychopathology: A guide for clinicians. *Journal of Psychoeducational Assessment, 25,* 139–149.

Tarnopolsky, A., Hand, D. J., McLean, E. K., Roberts, H., & Wiggins, R. D. (1979). Validity and uses of a screening questionnaire (GHQ) in the community. *British Journal of Psychiatry, 134,* 508–515.

VanDeventer, M. C. (2008). Universal emotional and behavioral screening for children and adolescents. Unpublished doctoral dissertation.

Vannest, K. J. (2012). Implementing interventions and progress monitoring subsequent to universal screening. *School Psychology Forum, 6*(4), 119–136.

Vannest, K. J., Reynolds, C. R., & Kamphaus, R. W. (2008). *BASC-2: Intervention guide.* Circle Pines: Pearson.

Walker, B. A. (2010). Effective schoolwide screening to identify students at risk for social and behavioral Problems. *Intervention in School and Clinic, 46,* 104–110.

Walker, H. M., & McConnell, S. R. (1995). *Walker-McConnell scale of social competence and school adjustment, elementary version: User's manual.* San Diego: Singular Publishing Group, Inc.

Walker, H. M., & Severson, H. H. (1992). *Systematic screening for behavior disorders (SSBD).* Longmont: Sopris West.

Walker, H. M., Small, J. W., Severson, H. H., Seeley, J. R., & Feil, E. G. (2014). Multiple-gating approaches in universal screening within school and community settings. In R. J. Kettler, T. A. Glover, C. A. Albers, & K. A. Feeney-Kettler (Eds.), *Universal screening in educational settings: Evidence-based decision making for schools* (pp. 47–75). Washington, DC: American Psychological Association.

Wallace, J. M., Goodkind, S., Wallace, C. M., & Bachman, J. G. (2008). Racial, ethnic, and gender differences in school discipline among U.S. high school students: 1991–2005. *Negro Education Review, 59*(1–2), 47–62.

Winter, L. B., Steer, R. A., Jones-Hicks, L., & Beck, A. T. (1999). Screening for major depression disorders in adolescent medical outpatients with the Beck Depression Inventory for primary care. *Journal of Adolescent Health, 24,* 389–394.

World Health Organization. (1993). *The ICD-10 classification of mental and behavioural disorders: Diagnostic criteria for research. World Health Organization.* Geneva: Author.

Yates, T., Ostroskly, M. M., Cheatham, G. A., Fettig, A., Shaffer, L., & Santos, R. M. (2008). Research synthesis on screening and assessing social-emotional competence. The Center on the Social and Emotional Foundations for Early Learning. Retrieved from Vanderbilt.edu/csefel.

Youngstrom, E., Loeber, R., & Stouthamer-Loeber, M. (2000). Patterns and correlates of agreement between parent, teacher, and male adolescent ratings of externalizing and internalizing problems. *Journal of Consulting and Clinical Psychology, 68,* 1038–1050.

Index

M. C. Stiffler, B. V. Dever, *Mental Health Screening at School*, Contemporary Issues in Psychological Assessment, DOI 10.1007/978-3-319-19171-3

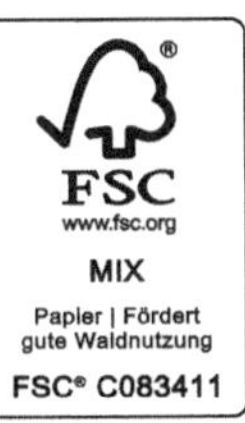

Zeitfracht Medien GmbH
Ferdinand-Jühlke-Straße 7
99095 Erfurt, Deutschland
produktsicherheit@kolibri360.de